GET
THROUGH

MRCGP
Clinical Skills Assessment

GET THROUGH

MRCGP
Clinical Skills Assessment

Second edition

Bruno Rushforth MA(Cantab) MBChB MA MRCGP DRCOG DFSRH
PG Cert Primary Care Ed
GP and Clinical Research Fellow in Primary Care
University of Leeds

Adam Firth BSc MBChB DTM&H DipPalMed MRES MRCGP
NIHR Academic Clinical Fellow in General Practice
The University of Manchester

Val Wass BSc FRCGP FRCP MHPE PhD
Professor of Medical Education and Head of Keele School of Medicine

CRC Press
Taylor & Francis Group
Boca Raton London New York

CRC Press is an imprint of the
Taylor & Francis Group, an **informa** business

First published in Great Britain in 2008 by the Royal Society of Medicine Press Ltd, UK
This second edition published in 2013 by
CRC Press
Taylor & Francis Group
6000 Broken Sound Parkway NW, Suite 300
Boca Raton, FL 33487-2742

CRC Press is an imprint of Taylor & Francis Group, an Informa business
No claim to original U.S. Government works
Version Date: 20120813
International Standard Book Number: 978-1-4441-6824-2
1 2 3 4 5 6 7 8 9 10

Visit the Taylor & Francis Web site at
http://www.taylorandfrancis.com
and the CRC Press Web site at
http://www.crcpress.com

Printed and bound by CPI Group (UK) Ltd, Croydon, CR0 4YY

CONTENTS

FOREWORD

When I read the first edition of this book I was impressed by the way that the authors had helped young doctors, studying to become general practitioners, understand the complexity of the consultation whilst preparing for the Clinical Skills Assessment of the MRCGP examination. The second edition builds on the delightful approach of the successful first edition with new scenarios and explanations of how to approach clinical situations in general practice and how to think holistically about patient care in first contact situations.

The book begins with an explanation of the MRCGP CSA and makes suggestions as to how best to prepare for it, throughout the year and in the days and hours before the assessment. This is followed by thirty two sections, each of which is intended to represent a station in the CSA. The scenarios cover a range of common situations encountered in general practice and offer a complete revision guide with advice on current best practice.

The authors encourage the learner to think about different settings and how they would approach the presenting problem; readers are encouraged to consider what might lie behind the presenting problem and how they might use their interpersonal skills effectively. They are also encouraged to think beyond the clinical example, reflecting on how, by changing one piece of information, a doctor might take a different approach to similar presenting symptoms. The book could be used for individual study or revision, but has been written in a way that also encourages peer learning and reflection and would be particularly useful as a basis for group study or for trainers to use with a range of learners in their practice, helping each to understand complex clinical management.

This edition continues to give insight into the thought processes of our examiners and it encourages a holistic approach to study rather than a 'box-ticking' approach or rote learning. It approaches the CSA positively and encourages trainees to think about the domains that need to be assessed (and demonstrated) to assure the public of fitness for completion of training. This edition raises the concept of 'red flags' and the importance or recognising less common but very significant pointers of serious conditions. I particularly liked another new concept: practising a one-minute explanation of issues encountered in the section. A simple but effective concept and one that could be used alone, video-recorded or in group learning.

I am certain that the second edition will be as popular as the first; helping trainers, their registrars and foundation trainees understand and explain the complexities of patient care in general practice.

Jacky Hayden

Dean of Postgraduate Medical Studies

North Western Deanery and University of Manchester

FOREWORD

This edition is also aimed at Family Doctors [as General Practitioners are more commonly known outside of the UK] who are preparing to undertake and pass the MRCGP [INT] examination for the country, or region of the world, where they work.

We know that, in spite of the wide variety of contexts in which Family Doctors work worldwide, differing because of the health systems, culture, epidemiology, language, history and geography, that at least two thirds of what we do is recognisably similar, while a third is locally specific. These similarities and differences are acknowledged in the differing curricula for the locally devised MRCGP [INT] examination sites in the Middle East, South Asia, South East Asia Pacific, North Africa and Europe.

In the West the ethos of patient-centred consulting has only become widely established for the past thirty years, with the international evidence for this collated in the last twenty years and then actively promoted by the World Organisation of Family Doctors [WONCA] and World Health Organisation [WHO]. The Royal College of General Practitioners successfully introduced this ethos into the UK curriculum firstly by means of establishing a video assessment of consulting skills into the MRCGP examination, which effected tremendous behavioural and cultural changes in GPs as well as more systematic analysis of the doctor–patient interaction.

Assessment can therefore drive the learning and the teaching. In a similar fashion, international pioneers of Family Medicine have developed local curricula and examinations to assess these, which the Royal College have successfully accredited with the MRCGP [INT], having similar academic rigour to the UK orientated MRCGP. These curricula have also recognised the evidence base for the emphasis on patient centred consulting and this is reflected in the various communication and clinical skills assessments that the differing MRCGP [INT] examination sites use, increasingly in the locally used language.

As this book emphasises, unless this ethos and the communication skills that underpin this are introduced into your own everyday work, merely rehearsing the learnt phrases for the examination will not be enough for you to succeed in passing the clinical skills examination for the MRCGP [INT]. The examiners can see where this ethos has been integrated into a candidate's own practice by the fluency, familiarity and personal approach in their interaction with the simulated patients of the examination.

This book suggests opportunities for you to think imaginatively how the scenarios may be applied to your own country, health system and culture. Furthermore, it encourages you to break down the defensive professional boundaries that we have, by suggesting that you identify and work with like minded colleagues, using the scenarios to rehearse what may initially feel are unfamiliar attitudes and language.

Feedback from very many successful MRCGP [INT] candidates has demonstrated how much integrating this approach has improved their own patient care and professional development, which their patients, community and professional colleagues will also recognise.

John V Howard FRCGP FRCP

Medical Director, MRCGP [INT] Programme

Royal College of General Practitioners

ACKNOWLEDGEMENTS

We would like to thank the following individuals for giving helpful feedback on earlier drafts of scenarios that we have subsequently updated from the first edition: Amy Evans, Rafik Taijbee, Wendy Brown, Nicola Cooper, Nat Wright, Jacki Barson, Linda Cusick, John Hamlin and Amy Grundy. Constructive comments on the new scenarios and updates for the second edition were kindly provided by Michael Bennett and Amy Evans. We are particularly indebted to the MRCGP[INT] South Asia team for the insight they have provided into the needs of candidates sitting International assessments.

The editorial team at Hodder Education has been supportive throughout and we are particularly grateful to Hannah Applin, Sarah Penny and Stephen Clausard for guiding us through the process of producing the second edition.

We thank the individuals and publishing bodies that gave permission for us to reproduce extracts from their work. All are credited in the text.

Finally, we are very grateful to Arja Kajermo for her observant and witty illustrations.

PREPARING FOR THE CLINICAL SKILLS ASSESSMENT: THE 'WHY', 'WHAT', 'WHEN' AND 'HOW'

This introduction outlines the Clinical Skills Assessment (CSA) and offers a strategy for revision. We consider 'why' there needs to be a skills test, and discuss 'what' it involves and 'when' to apply to take it. Advice on 'how' to use this book to prepare for the CSA is then given. For this second edition we have expanded the focus. The book has found an increasing market with readers beyond the UK preparing for Membership of the Royal College of General Practitioners [International] (MRCGP[INT]) clinical skills assessments. We offer advice on preparation for candidates who have qualified abroad and are less familiar with the UK setting and for those preparing for International examinations, which use simulated patients.

Why a clinical skills assessment?

Formal examinations have come under increasing scrutiny now that it is acknowledged that assessment on performance in the workplace – i.e. what a doctor actually *does* – is the gold standard to aim for. The MRCGP UK is no exception. There is now considerable emphasis on the e-portfolio of workplace-based assessment tasks that need to be completed throughout GP specialty training, supported by discussion and formative review with your trainer.

So why have an examination as well? The reasons are perhaps self-evident. We cannot yet be assured that assessments of performance are robust. The range of cases covered using the workplace-based tools will vary widely across different placements. The challenge of the tasks will differ, as will the quality of judgements made by assessors. From the patient's perspective, the e-portfolio alone cannot assure a licensing body that the training curriculum has been covered. Yet candidates in the past have not always felt that their trainer has been fair. This can be difficult in the one-to-one supervision offered by general practice. Inevitably, examinations must stay. If approached in the right way, they offer a positive opportunity to consolidate the skills learned through consistent practice during training and through regular contact with patients.

We cannot emphasize too strongly the importance of applying to take the CSA only when you feel secure that you have developed the necessary skills through everyday contact with patients in the cultural context of the country in which you practise. Assessment is changing. There is an increasing understanding that the methods selected to assess trainees must complement each other. The results need to be compared and integrated to ensure that a full and accurate perspective of the candidate's ability and level of performance is obtained. It is important to recognize this when studying for the CSA. Do not approach it in isolation as separate from the Applied Knowledge Test (AKT) or from your e-portfolio.

The applied evidence-based knowledge tested in the AKT is essential to your performance in the CSA to demonstrate, for example, that you can use guidelines to reach appropriate management decisions.

Formative assessments for the e-portfolio and/or group sessions with peers working towards the formal accreditation should be planned to inform your preparation. Identical patient-centred, evidence-based, shared management structures underpin all components of the MRCGP assessments. Workplace-based assessment and/or peer observation present ideal opportunities to get feedback on areas you are concerned about. Harness the thinking behind the MRCGP to your advantage.

View the CSA as part of an assessment package. Do not study for it in isolation.

Tips for preparation for the CSA

- Ensure that you actively practise in the context in which the CSA is set. It is important to understand cultural values even in a simulated setting.
- Integrate preparation with your e-portfolio or keep a reflective diary of your daily work.
- Log your consultations. Identify gaps for revision against the curriculum.
- Video your consultations from early on and discuss these regularly with your trainer and/or peers.
- Harness formative assessments with your trainer to develop your CSA skills.
- Prepare carefully for case-based discussions using the suggested framework.
- Use COT (Consultation Observation Tool) and DOPS (Direct Observation of Procedural Skills) assessments to get feedback on all the listed clinical skills.
- Reflect at the end of every surgery. Identify areas for improvement.
- Make notes on consultations to use for revision and practise with colleagues.
- If you have not trained with simulated patients, use role-play with your supervisor and peers repeatedly to practise.
- Write your own scenarios for role-play based on actual consultations and the expanded tasks we have developed for this second edition.

What is the CSA?

The CSA assesses a '*demonstration*' of how you work when consulting in the surgery. You are invited to show the examiners how you would manage a range of simulated consultation scenarios in real life. If you prepare inadequately there is the danger of artificial rather than authentic performance. You should not rely on short preparation courses. The patient-centred skills required of clinical skills assessments cannot be learned this way.

In the past you may have revised for undergraduate Objective Structured Clinical Examinations (OSCEs) by memorizing checklists for the skills under test, grooming these on preparation courses or using books such as this one. Your rehearsed behaviours may not have related to your usual practice. Indeed, it has been argued that clinical tests can make 'monkeys of men', producing 'tick list' performances which score highly but are not at all reflective of actual practice. This can lead to faked behaviours and artificial performance. Preparation for this examination must be strategic and practice based to avoid this pitfall. Relying on preparation courses is not enough and misleading. The skills you require are embedded in your actual practice and can be learned only through face-to-face contact with real patients.

So why does the MRCGP use an OSCE-type format? Do not be misled. This is a postgraduate examination and different. Clinical skills tests of general practice have been designed to test an integrated approach to the consultation based on real-life experiences. There is no checklist to perform against or expectation of perfect performance. Your approach should mirror that of daily practice, i.e. patient-centred consultations resulting in safe and appropriate shared management decisions. The assessment is designed to be as authentic as possible. We deliberately offer full, detailed scenarios that reflect the complexity of everyday encounters. The challenge is to work with the scenarios and practise reaching shared management decisions within the timed framework of the CSA. There is no ideal model answer.

> Prepare in everyday practice: aim for authentic not artificial performance.

Familiarity with a wide range of common presenting problems is essential across patients of different age, gender, ethnicity and social class. It is important to understand the cultural context of UK practice. Herein lies a significant difficulty for doctors trained abroad. Health beliefs, cultural understanding and the National Health Service (NHS) structure itself are imperceptibly bound into the consultation. This is why, in contrast to other UK Royal Colleges, the RCGP does not export the UK examination to other countries. Candidates from abroad found the old UK MRCGP difficult to pass as they were unfamiliar with the UK context. General practice consultations depend on the local population mix, which in some practices may not reflect the full breadth of experience required by the CSA. We recommend that you discuss this with your trainer and ensure that you acquire the necessary familiarity with UK patients before you sit the CSA.

Arrange to observe peers in other practices and, if necessary, ensure you consult in a range of settings. The scenarios in this book have been written to reflect the breadth of contexts you might meet in the CSA. Tasks have been introduced to enable you to explore more widely the various ways a patient might present and offer different permutations for practise. For those sitting International examinations we suggest ways to modify the scenarios to address the local context of their work.

The set-up

The UK CSA consists of 13 standardized simulated consultations that test your ability to integrate consultation and clinical skills or consult with other professionals within the primary care team at an appropriate level of challenge. Each consultation is 10 minutes with a 2-minute break in between. The examination is structured to allow you to feel you are sitting in a surgery with the simulated patient entering (accompanied by the examiner) to consult with you. Focus on the patient and ignore the examiner.

> Observe your surroundings carefully on arrival: note the available equipment.

To embrace the full context of primary care the stations may include a telephone consultation and/or home visit. In the 2-minute break between patients you may be taken to a telephone which rings at the start of the station, allowing you to consult with the simulated patient who is placed out of sight accompanied by the examiner. Alternatively, you may be taken into a room 'mocked up' as the patient's house. At the end of this station you return to your consultation room.

Dress as you would for formal professional practice, ensuring you respect the simulators as though they were real patients. At the same time be aware that the examiners expect your appearance to be compatible with your professional role and will be assessing your non-verbal as well as your verbal behaviour. We recommend that you read the advice offered by the RCGP on dress code.

Recommended equipment for your doctor's bag

You will be asked to bring a doctor's bag of basic equipment with you. Below is a summary of what this should include. Remember to take it with you if you move stations for a home visit consultation.

British National Formulary (BNF)
Stethoscope
Ophthalmoscope
Auroscope
Thermometer
Patella hammer
Peak flow meter and disposable mouth pieces (N.B. These must be European Union standard)
Tape measure

The *BNF* cannot be annotated and you are not allowed to take any other equipment into the consultation room. Any additional items that might be required will be provided at the assessment centre. When you arrive, you will be asked to transfer your equipment to a clear plastic wallet before the exam begins.

The consultation process

There will be a set of basic notes for each consultation in a folder on the desk to read in the break between consultations.

> Read the patient information carefully, trying to formulate what is being tested.

A buzzer will sound to mark the beginning and end of each station. After the first buzzer, the patient will knock on the door or just enter, accompanied by an examiner. There are clocks in all rooms to help you judge the time. The consultation ends as soon as the second buzzer sounds – you cannot score any additional marks after this point. The simulated patient has been trained against a written script and the content can be covered in the allocated time. The tricky part is deciding whether a physical examination and/or clinical procedure (e.g. peak flow) are required. The examiner may guide you, but do not rely on this. This is the only point in the process where they may interact. If you feel an intimate examination is indicated, you can suggest this, although it should not be attempted unless a model is provided. If you say that you would like to examine the patient, there are three possibilities:

- The patient may simply give you a card with the examination findings.
- The examiner may intervene and state, for example, 'Assume the chest is clear'.
- You will be required to carry out the appropriate examination and given any findings at the end.

The patient may simply give you a card with the examination findings. The examiner may intervene and state, for example, 'Assume the chest is clear'. You will be required to carry out the appropriate examination and given any findings at the end.

This emphasizes the importance of the workplace-based assessments, e.g. COTs, in developing appropriate focused examinations through being observed and receiving feedback. Remember to gain consent for any examination and to explain the procedure to the patient.

Practise focused physical examinations using the workplace-based tools.

The marking system

The examiner silently makes an overall judgement in three performance domains of your ability:

Domain 1: Interpersonal skills. Integrate eliciting the patient's agenda and understanding of the problem with the specific information needed to make a diagnosis and shared decisions. Scenarios are designed to assess your ability to handle a range of patient emotions, display ethical practice and demonstrate respect for equality and diversity.

Domain 2: Data gathering, technical and assessment skills. Elicit the appropriate information needed to make a clinical judgement on the patient's presenting problem, decide whether a physical examination is required and undertake this, supplementing it with other clinical procedures where appropriate.

Domain 3: Clinical management skills. Recognize and manage common presenting complaints in general practice. These include undifferentiated problems, multiple complaints and issues that require a holistic approach to promote healthy living. You are expected to demonstrate a flexible, evidence-based and structured approach to decision making with patients.

An overall mark for each station is then given: clear pass, pass, fail or clear fail. Examiners are trained and have guidelines to standardize marking. However, they are making 'global' rather than 'checklist' judgements. They are assessing your overall, integrated approach to the consultation, not ticking off a list of observed behaviours. The more experience you have gained in the surgery with your trainer, the more expert and natural your performance will be. Familiarity with a wide range of common presenting problems is essential across patients of different age, gender, ethnicity and social class. Only practice in the workplace will achieve this. We cannot emphasize enough the intentions of this marking system.

When should you take the CSA?

This is a matter for you and your trainer but it should take place in ST3 at a point when you have both a sound knowledge base and a fluent, culturally appropriate, patient-centred consultation style. You must be able to apply guidelines using evidence-based practice and have sound diagnostic and consultation skills. Exploring the patient's agenda fully and formulating a shared patient plan must emerge naturally within your consultation. This requires experience and training using video feedback with your trainer and peers. You need to be well grounded in practice. The examination may feel like 'the surgery from hell', but you should have the experience to feel 'this is like being at work'. You should also have mastered the knowledge base needed for general practice.

How does this book support you in preparing for the CSA?

This second edition of the book offers 32 stations, each with notes. We have designed a revision strategy to build a framework for your preparation. This aims to help you transfer skills from everyday practice into the simulated context of the examination. The notes after each scenario offer ideal approaches that cannot necessarily be covered fully in 10 minutes. We have aimed to paint a full picture. Remember, the examiners are not looking for perfect consultations but a sound, integrated, well-informed and patient-centred approach. Failing to cover all three domains and reach a shared management outcome with the patient is one of the most common reasons for failing. We have structured the scenarios to encourage you to address the areas where candidates commonly have difficulty. The following table summarizes the behaviours the examiners are looking for and how this book supports you in achieving these.

Positive behaviours the examiners are looking for	How to use this book to achieve this
Approaches logically and sequentially: no non-sequential after thoughts	Practise permutations of the scenarios and tasks within the CSA time frame
Uses open questions to identify the patient's agendas	Make notes of your expectations before and after you read the scenarios
Uses open to closed questions to gather data and reach a diagnosis	The scenarios illustrate what simulated patients will deliver freely or not
Addresses the patient's health beliefs and preferences	Opportunities to adapt to international practice
Listens actively to pick up cues fluently	Emphasizes need to learn this through real-life practice
Explains in language a patient can understand	Practise the I-minute explanations and invent your own
Competent physical examination and use of instruments	Scenarios identify which examinations are appropriate in the CSA setting
Achieves an appropriate differential diagnosis	Content illustrates and gives essential knowledge for common problems

(continued)

Positive behaviours the examiners are looking for	How to use this book to achieve this
Achieves a management plan based on the current evidence base	All scenarios have updated information on current evidence-based practice
Applies current NHS practice and governance to management	NHS context emphasized throughout with suggestions extended for non-UK candidates
Makes patients aware of management options and risks	Scenarios contain opportunities to do this with information to assess risk
Addresses health promotion issues wherever relevant	Opportunities to do this are embedded in the wide range of scenarios
Concludes with follow-up and safety-netting arrangements	Use the scenarios to ensure you can achieve this within 9–10 minutes
Manages the time to reach a shared management decision	The detailed scenarios enable different approaches and permutations

After reading the notes, re-run the scenarios, aiming to cover all three domains within 9 minutes at a 'realistic' but not 'perfect' level. We must stress the importance of reaching a shared management conclusion within the time allocated. Aim to do this well within the 9 minutes. This we feel allows for the anxiety that might delay you a little in the real examination. We have added tasks to enable you to explore different patient agendas and, for MRCGP[INT] candidates, to adapt to your own cultural family medicine context. We are also aware that examiners are looking for clear, effective explanations to patients to underpin shared management decisions. We have added suggestions for specific areas where you might like to practise giving 'lay' explanations in the constricted time frame you will experience in the CSA. Ask colleagues to observe and check that you use language a patient will understand. In addition to the cases in this book, try writing your own scenarios based on patients you see in surgery. Check the knowledge on which management decisions should be based and then offer them to colleagues for practice. The CSA is written from everyday examples and you will find you can do this just as well.

We strongly recommend that you prepare with a group of peers. Candidates trained in non-UK medical schools may not be familiar with role-play. If this is the case, ensure that you practise in a group that includes UK-trained peers who are familiar with learning through role-play and can help you adapt to this as a learning method. Try to gain experience of working with professional role-players as well. Opportunities may arise during your vocational training day-release sessions. If not, discuss the need with your trainer and ensure that you gain some experience in doing this.

We have structured the scenarios in the book to illustrate how the role-player's script can influence the consultation. They are trained to deliver information with open questioning followed by specific questioning. Keeping the simulated consultation 'open' at the start is therefore essential to gain as much information as possible before you ask more specific questions (see below, Step 3). This, of course, reflects real life and the importance of eliciting the patient's agenda in your day-to-day work in the surgery. However, role-play does feel different alongside the time pressures of the CSA consultation and we recommend that you become familiar with this practice, which is now used extensively in UK medical schools for communication skills training.

Step 1: Build a revision framework from the two test grids (see Appendices 1 and 2)

The scope of the curriculum is large. It is important that you revisit this regularly on the RCGP website (www.rcgp.org.uk). We have designed grids to illustrate.

The skills being tested are devised from the marking criteria:

Category of skill

Gender mix	Age mix	Skills in diagnosis	Ongoing management skills	Clinical practical skills	Health promotion	Diversity and ethical issues	Dealing with patients' emotions

The contexts of common presentations that will be covered based on the curriculum.

Key for test grids: contexts covered based on the curriculum

Cardiovascular problems (CVD)
Digestive problems (GI)
Ear, nose and throat, and facial problems (ENT)
Eye problems (Eye)
Metabolic problems (Endo)
Neurological problems (Neuro)
Respiratory problems (Resp)
Rheumatology, musculoskeletal and trauma (Rheum)
Skin problems (Derm)
Genetics in primary care (Gene)
Care of acutely ill people (Acute)
Care of children and young people (Paed)
Care of older adults (Geri)
Women's health (F)
Men's health (M)
Sexual health (Sex)
Care of people with cancer and palliative care (Pall)
Care of people with mental health problems (Psy)
Drug and alcohol problems (Drug use)
Healthy people: promoting health and preventing disease (H Pro)
Care of people with learning disabilities (Learn dis)

We suggest that you build a portfolio of consultations in your practice using these grids to identify the gaps in presentation and management that you need to cover before sitting the CSA.

Develop a grid to plot your consultations; identify gaps for revision.

Step 2: Build a framework to formulate what the simulated consultation is testing

On first reading the station instructions to candidates, we encourage you to jot down, in the space provided, your initial thoughts on what is being tested before you read on. Commit yourself to doing this in anticipation of doing this in the CSA itself.

The full simulated patient scenario is then included to illustrate the importance of eliciting a comprehensive patient narrative to fully assess the purpose of the station. If you do not do this, key areas may be missed.

Practise eliciting full patient narratives to ensure that you don't miss hidden agendas.

Step 3: Work with the simulated patient

The simulated patient script has an additional purpose. Just as in real life a patient presents with a narrative (and we have encouraged you to record the ones you encounter in practice), so does the simulated patient. In the CSA these scenarios have been scripted to give the information needed to formulate diagnoses and management plans in the areas being tested. The simulated patient is not going to play 'cat and mouse' as patients sometimes unwittingly do. The information you require is in front of you, waiting to be elicited. Ask open questions and the simulated patient can respond only as scripted. Responses to direct closed questions are also highlighted to illustrate the integration of data gathering into the interview. We use the scenario to highlight that it is crucial to listen sensitively in the initial phases of the consultation. Look for non-verbal cues as well. For example, in one station offered in this book, the patient has a packet of cigarettes in his breast pocket.

The simulated patient has a script to deliver: use open questions initially to elicit this.

Keep up to date with management guidelines: identify and 'plug' knowledge gaps.

Step 4: Identify the full range of outcomes the examiner is looking for

After reading the patient's script, pause again and review what you now think the station is assessing. Again, there is space provided for you to make notes. We strongly recommend that you do this. You should be able to formulate the issues the examiner is looking for under the headings: interpersonal skills, data gathering and clinical management. Then move on. The discussion section gives our expectations, which you can compare with your notes and discuss with colleagues. Remember, you are aiming for sensible yet fluent coverage, not necessarily the ideal fully comprehensive scenario set out in the book.

Aim in the 10 minutes to formulate a sensible, fluent outcome: it will not be perfect.

Step 5: Your knowledge base

It is important to keep reviewing and updating your reading. It is a mistake to view skills as distinct from knowledge. It is of paramount importance to patients that the information given and management decisions made are grounded in up-to-date, evidence-based practice. We have outlined how each station links with the preparation you require for the AKT. The information is detailed. We acknowledge that you cannot necessarily cover it all in 10 minutes. The aim is to illustrate how everyday practice can structure reading and revision for the CSA.

Use the book to develop your own scenarios for group revision.

Step 6: Write your own stations

We have aimed to offer a framework for doing this and ideas for further revision. Scenarios can be adapted to work with colleagues or alternative ones written.

Step 7: Finally

Why have so many stations if the marking schedule is a generic one? Herein lies a basic principle of assessment that has an important practical message. Doctors are not consistent in their practice. We are all good in some contexts and not so good in others. Inevitably, however well prepared, you will perform better on some stations than others. It is crucial that you can handle this. If you feel that you have done badly on a consultation, avoid using the 2-minute break to reflect on this. Keep thinking forwards and focus immediately on the instructions for the next station, where you may well perform brilliantly.

   We wish you well. Good luck.

Think forwards in the CSA, not backwards: some stations will be better than others.

Summary

Study the curriculum	Regularly review the curriculum. Keep up to date and evidence based. Make a grid to identify revision needs
Understand the skills	Develop well-integrated clinical competencies. Do not work from checklists. Get feedback through direct observation or using video. Harness workplace-based assessments
Practise the skills	The more experience the better, across a range of common presentations and a diversity of patients
Work with your peers	Revise together. Develop scenarios from everyday practice. Observe, role-play, give feedback. It can be fun!
Use the CSA format	Use the breaks to think forwards, keep your eyes open, listen effectively and keep to the patient-centred, shared-management structure throughout
Remain confident	Develop the right mentality. You will undoubtedly 'flunk' some stations. Learn to move confidently on to the next

Information given to candidates

Wendy Morrison is a 30-year-old mother-of-two who works as an administrator and rarely sees her doctor. You note that her records show one episode of depression 6 years ago, which resolved without the need for medication or referral.

She saw one of the other GPs in the practice last week complaining of feeling tired all the time. Physical examination was normal and urine dip-stick was negative.

The results of her blood tests taken last week are:

Haemoglobin (Hb)	12.8 g/L	(12.0–15.0)	Thyroid-stimulating hormone (TSH)	2.12 mIU/L	(0.35–5.5)
White cell count (WCC)	7.5 × 10⁹/L	(4.0–11.0)	T4	18 pmol/L (8–22)	
Platelets	258 × 10⁹/L	(150–400)			
Na	138 mmol/L	(135–145)	Glucose	5.0 mmol/L	(4.0–6.0)
K	4.2 mmol/L	(3.5–5.0)			
Urea	4.2 mmol/L	(3.0–6.5)			
Creatinine	82 µmol/L	(60–125)			

As you open the consultation the patient begins to cry and says that she feels so low she 'just can't go on'.

- What do you think this station is testing?
- Make notes or discuss your thoughts with a colleague before you read on.

Plan your approach to this station:

Information given to simulated patient

Basic details – You are Wendy Morrison, a Caucasian 30-year-old female administrator.

Appearance and behaviour – You begin to cry after the GP opens the consultation. However, you soon recover your composure. You are well presented and maintain good eye contact during the consultation.

History

Freely divulged to doctor – You have been feeling low, slowed down and tired all the time for about 4 months. You are sleeping badly – finding it hard to get off to sleep and in the last month you have also been waking up at about 5 am and cannot get back to sleep, even though you feel exhausted.

Divulged to doctor if specifically asked – You were working 3 days a week but went full-time 6 months ago as money was tight and you and your husband are saving for a deposit on a house. Since then you have been finding it difficult to cope with the demands of running the home, looking after the children and working full-time. Your husband is sympathetic but is out at work himself much of the time. You had to give up your weekly get-together with friends as you just did not have the time to spare. You now find it hard to concentrate on things and your appetite is poor. You cannot seem to get any enjoyment out of the things you used to like, such as watching TV or reading. In the last week you have felt that you cannot go on like this, but you have never thought of hurting yourself in any way and have no such current thoughts of self-harm or suicide. You have never tried to hurt yourself in the past. You took today off work – your first day sick in 3 years – but told work that you had the flu. You came to see the doctor last week to say all this, but felt 'stupid' so did not mention your mood.

Ideas, concerns and expectations – You see yourself as a 'coper' and your family and friends describe you as a 'rock' in supporting them with all their problems. You feel 'weak' not being able to get well by yourself, and have put off coming to see the doctor. You have not told any family or friends that you are here today as you are embarrassed at seeking help for something that you think you should just 'snap out of'. However, you are frightened that your mood seems to be worse than when you were depressed 6 years ago. You are also worried at being labelled with a mental health problem and particularly do not want work to find out. You are hoping that the blood results will show some physical problem to explain your symptoms. If you need treatment for your low mood then you would prefer a 'natural' remedy, such as St John's wort, rather than prescription tablets, but you want to talk to the doctor and find out more about this. You think 'counselling' with a 'stranger' would be a waste of time.

First words spoken to doctor – 'I'm sorry, doctor, but I feel so low I just can't go on.'

Medical history – After the birth of your second child you felt low and tearful for several weeks and saw the doctor twice about this (on your mother's insistence). Things got better on their own and you put it down to the 'baby blues' and thought no more about it. You rarely see the doctor and have attended previously for pill checks and cervical smears.

Drug history – You are not allergic to any medication. You take the combined contraceptive pill – Microgynon 30.

Social history – You live with your husband and two sons – aged 6 and 8 – in a large rented flat. Your husband works as a self-employed shop-fitter. Your mother lives nearby and looks after the children after school. You drink the occasional glass of wine at home with meals. You have never smoked.

Family history – There is no history of mental health problems in your family.

- Having read the information given to the simulated patient, what do you now think this station is testing?
- Make notes or discuss your thoughts with a colleague before you turn the page.

Review your approach to this station:

Tested at this station:

1. Dealing with a distressed patient.
2. Understanding a patient's illness experience.
3. Taking a depression history.
4. Self-harm risk assessment.
5. Reaching a shared management plan.
6. Appropriate follow-up and safety netting.

Domain I – Interpersonal skills

Dealing with a distressed patient

This patient is visibly upset. You need to spend the first part of the consultation quickly building an empathic, trusting relationship and exploring her distress:

- Allow the patient to speak uninterrupted and employ active listening skills such as non-verbal communication to demonstrate your interest and concern.
- Use silences to give the patient time to express her thoughts and feelings.
- Verbalize her distress – *'I can see that you're obviously upset'*.
- Paraphrase and summarize to demonstrate active listening and to help confirm your understanding.
- When a patient is upset, appropriate use of touch – e.g. on the arm – can act as a powerful show of support and empathy. However, this must be an authentic response to the situation rather than a forced move. Whether you choose to use it will depend on a number of factors, including the room set-up, the rapport between yourself and the patient, your judgement on how it will be received and whether you feel comfortable with such an act. If there is any doubt in your mind about the appropriateness of touch in any situation then it is best not to use it.
- The new GP curriculum talks about finding a balance between emotional distance and proximity to the patient – in other words, be caring but stay objective and professional.

Understanding a patient's illness experience (overlap with domain 2)

As medics, we are used to diagnostic categories, but these are the bare medical bones that you need to flesh out by building up a picture of the patient's illness experience:

- Open questions are most appropriate to begin with to elicit the patient's story and help you understand the patient's unique perspective.
- Explore the patient's ideas, concerns and expectations. How is her life affected by these problems? What are her thoughts about what is making her feel like this? What most worries her about the current situation? Why did she not mention her mood last week when she saw your colleague? What does she want from seeing you today?

Domain 2 – Data gathering, technical and assessment skills

Taking a depression history

Hopefully you will have obtained much relevant information from your initial open questions. However, you may need to follow this up with some more specific enquiries:

- Ask about mood, sleep, appetite, concentration, anhedonia (loss of capacity to experience pleasure), feelings of guilt, hopelessness and helplessness, and time off work.
- What support structures are in place to help her through this difficult time – friends, family, work?
- Does she have any anxiety symptoms? Depression and anxiety commonly co-exist.
- What has she tried to help? Does she feel anything has worked?
- What prescribed medication does she take? Remember that medication such as β-blockers can cause depression.
- You might also want to ask about alcohol and any illicit drug use, as these can affect mood or be used by patients as a coping strategy.
- What happened during the previous episode of depression? How do things now compare with then?

Self-harm risk assessment

For any patient presenting with depression you must undertake a risk assessment for deliberate self-harm, which includes suicide:

- Be sensitive when asking about this subject – wait for an appropriate point in the consultation when you have built up rapport.
- *'How low have you felt at your worst'* is a useful opening question.
- Do not shy away from asking a direct question about whether the patient has thought about harming herself or ending her life.
- Has she acted on any such thoughts – e.g. made plans, written notes to loved ones, arranged her financial affairs?
- Any previous suicide attempts or other self-harm?
- You already know about her medical history of depression, but have any close family members also had mental health problems?

Domain 3 – Clinical management skills

Reaching a shared management plan (overlap with domain 1)

From reading the simulated patient information you will see that this patient has her own perspective on mental health problems and thoughts about treatment options. You should have elicited these during the consultation and now attempt to incorporate her preferences when negotiating a shared management plan:

- Reassure her that the blood test results are normal. How does she feel about this?
- Ensure that you explain the diagnosis in simple, unambiguous terms. In this case it is *moderate depression*. What does she think of this?
- Explain how depression can affect things such as sleep, appetite and concentration. Does she have any questions about this?

- Present various management options. What are her thoughts on these? Any worries about any of the options? They might include:
  - General advice on self-help measures such as exercise and sleep hygiene.
  - Seeking social support from family and friends. Is there any way she could start going again to the weekly get-together of friends?
  - St John's wort – the patient initially appears in favour of this treatment, but is she fully informed about this option? Does she understand that although it can be effective in depression it has the potential to interact with other drugs and that it is difficult to know how much active treatment is present in certain preparations? Would you respect her wishes if, once fully informed, she still expressed a strong desire to self-medicate using St John's wort?
  - The National Institute for Health and Clinical Excellence (NICE) guidelines (see below) list anti-depressants as a treatment option for moderate depression. If she decides to try anti-depressants, check for any drug allergies before prescribing. Advise her that she might initially feel more anxious or agitated and that it may take a few weeks before she notices any improvement. Warn her of common side effects such as gastro-intestinal upset. Explain the potential withdrawal symptoms if she stops the tablets suddenly and that it is recommended to stay on the medication for at least 6 months after recovery.
  - 'Talking therapies' – e.g. cognitive behavioural therapy (CBT) with a therapist. What does she think of this?
  - Time off work – advise her that she can self-certify for the first 7 days, or if she wants you to write a sickness certificate for longer, you need to negotiate what to put down as the diagnosis. Is she happy for you to put 'depression' on the form?
- Would she like some written information such as a patient information leaflet on depression?
- Is the agreed plan mutually satisfactory, i.e. to patient and doctor?

Appropriate follow-up and safety netting

Negotiating appropriate follow-up and what to do if things deteriorate is essential for those patients presenting with depression:

- Discuss with the patient how she should be seen again in 2 weeks, or earlier if she prefers.
- Ask whether she would like the contact number of the local Mental Health Support Services. Let her know that she can call them anytime day or night if things get worse and she feels she needs immediate help.
- To make sure that follow-up arrangements have been fully understood you could ask the patient to describe the plan back to you.

Knowledge base – Stepped care management of depression

The stepped care model provides a framework in which to organize the provision of services, and supports patients, carers and practitioners in identifying and accessing the most effective interventions (see figure). In stepped care the least intrusive, most effective intervention is provided first. If a person does not benefit from the intervention initially offered, or declines an intervention, they should be offered an appropriate intervention from the next step.

Focus of the intervention	Nature of the intervention
STEP 4: Severe and complex[a] depression; risk to life; severe self-neglect	Medication, high-intensity psychological interventions, electroconvulsive therapy, crisis service, combined treatments, multiprofessional and inpatient care
STEP 3: Persistent subthreshold depressive symptoms or mild to moderate depression with inadequate response to initial interventions; moderate and severe depression	Medication, high-intensity psychological interventions, combined treatments, collaborative care[b] and referral for further assessment and intervention
STEP 2: Persistent subthreshold depressive symptoms; mild to moderate depression	Low-intensity psychosocial interventions, psychological interventions, medication and referral for further assessment and interventions
STEP 1: All known and suspected presentations of depression	Assessment, support, psychoeducation, active monitoring and referral for further assessment and interventions

[a] Complex depression includes depression that shows an inadequate response to multiple treatments, is complicated by psychotic symptoms, and/or is associated with significant psychiatric comorbidity or psychosocial factors.

[b] Only for depression where the person also has a chronic physical health problem and associated functional impairment (see 'Depression in adults with a chronic physical health problem: treatment and management' [NICE clinical guideline 91]).

The stepped care model. National Institute for Health and Clinical Excellence (NICE) (2009) CG 90 Depression: The treatment and management of depression in adults. London: NICE. Available from www.nice.org.uk/nicemedia/live/12329/45888/45888.pdf

---

Take-home messages

- How you relate to the patient – ideally showing respect and empathy at what is a difficult time for them – is more important than focusing your energies on an extensive checklist of questions.
- Risk assessment for deliberate self-harm must involve asking direct questions about thoughts of suicide.
- When negotiating a treatment plan, the key is to find out what the patient wants from coming to see the doctor.

Tasks

- Try re-running the scenario with the patient suffering from mild depression and willing to access computerized CBT.
- Try re-running the scenario with the patient suffering from severe depression with a high suicide risk.
- Try re-running the scenario with the patient's husband coming to discuss his concerns about the patient's mood.

1-minute explanations for patients

- Explain the CBT approach to managing depression.
- Counsel a patient about complementary and alternative medicine.
- Describe the biological model of depression.

Ideas for further revision

In primary care, patients regularly present in distress or can become tearful during the consultation. After each such consultation, take a few moments to reflect on what you felt went well, and what you might have done differently, to help you manage these emotionally charged encounters.

Further reading

NHS Clinical Knowledge Summaries: depression www.cks.nhs.uk/depression

NICE guidelines – Depression: The treatment and management of depression in adults. Clinical guidelines 90. October 2009 www.nice.org.uk

RCGP curriculum statement 13 – Care of people with mental health problems www.rcgp.org.uk

STATION 2

Information given to candidates

Steven Pinner is a 54-year-old electrician with asthma who failed to respond to two previous requests to see the practice nurse for an asthma review. His records state that he gave up smoking 20 years ago.

In the last 3 months he has had three repeat prescriptions for his salbutamol inhaler and four repeat prescriptions for his beclometasone inhaler.

He attended the local emergency department last week and the discharge sheet reads:

Patient: Steven Pinner

Attended St Benedict's emergency department complaining of 3-day history of

- *wheeze*
- *worsening shortness of breath*
- *chest tightness.*

On arrival peak expiratory flow rate (PEFR) = 360 L/min (patient does not know best; predicted 590 L/min)

No features of acute severe asthma

Electrocardiogram (ECG) – sinus tachycardia

Chest x-ray – no abnormalities seen, awaiting formal reporting

Diagnosis – moderate asthma attack

Treated with O_2, nebulized salbutamol and oral steroids

PEFR post nebulizer = 520 L/min

Symptoms resolved, therefore discharged with 5-day course of prednisolone 40 mg OD

To see GP for follow-up

As the patient enters the consulting room you note that he has a packet of cigarettes in his shirt pocket.

- What do you think this station is testing?
- Make notes or discuss your thoughts with a colleague before you read on.

Plan your approach to this station:

Information given to simulated patient

Basic details – You are Steven Pinner, a Caucasian 54-year-old male electrician.

Appearance and behaviour – You have a packet of cigarettes in the breast pocket of your shirt.

History

Freely divulged to doctor – Your breathing has been getting worse over the last 3 months. Your partner said that she could hear you wheezing when you arrived back from the corner shop. You know that this is probably because you have started smoking again. You went to the emergency department 5 days ago as you were finding it difficult to get your breath when you woke up one morning. They gave you oxygen and some medication through a mask. Your symptoms improved so you were sent home with a supply of steroid tablets (8 daily for 5 days).

Divulged to doctor if specifically asked – You did not make a conscious decision to start smoking again but just 'fell into it' when you moved in with your partner 3 months ago and this 'set off' your asthma. You were waking with a cough two or three times a night and you felt short of breath and wheezy climbing a flight of stairs. You have not coughed up any blood or phlegm, but your chest felt tight when the breathing was bad. You felt much better after having the treatment in hospital. Your breathing has been good since you were discharged and you went back to work 2 days after attending the hospital without any problems. You have cut down to about 10 cigarettes a day since leaving hospital. You meant to respond to the asthma nurse review letters but find it difficult to get time off work to attend appointments. You cannot remember the last time you had your peak flow checked or what it was. Twenty years ago a family friend who smoked heavily died of lung cancer and when you heard this you decided to quit smoking, which you did the same day without any help.

Ideas, concerns and expectations – You were frightened by the asthma attack last week as nothing like that has ever happened before. You were taking the steroid tablets given to you by the hospital at night but you felt they disturbed your sleep so you stopped taking them after 3 days (you had been told to take eight tablets each day for 5 days). You want to stop smoking but feel you need help with this, especially as your partner smokes but does not want to stop, and this is causing arguments at home. Since you started smoking again you have been thinking about the family friend who died of lung cancer and how you might go the same way if you don't quit. You did try to make an appointment to see the practice nurse who runs the smoking cessation clinic but you could not get through on the telephone. You are hoping that the doctor today will be able to give you some help with stopping smoking; you have heard about nicotine patches and gum.

First words spoken to doctor – 'The hospital said that I should come and see you about what happened.'

Medical history – You had keyhole surgery on your left knee 12 years ago to remove damaged cartilage after you slipped and fell. You have had antibiotics from the GP for chest infections on a couple of occasions over the last 5 years. Otherwise you are normally fit and well.

Drug history – You have two inhalers: a blue salbutamol inhaler and a brown beclometasone inhaler. You rarely used either of them until 3 months ago. Then you had been using them up to eight times a day each, but you don't really understand the difference between the two. You are not allergic to any medication. You have used the blue and brown inhalers only twice each since leaving hospital.

Social history – You are divorced from the mother of your two sons and had been living on your own for 5 years until you moved into your female partner's terraced house 3 months ago. You have been in the same job for more than 10 years. You drink 5 or 6 pints of beer over the weekend at the pub with friends.

Family history – You have two adult sons. Neither has asthma but one has eczema.

- Having read the information given to the simulated patient, what do you now think this station is testing?
- Make notes or discuss your thoughts with a colleague before you turn the page.

Review your approach to this station:

Tested at this station:

1. Understanding a patient's illness experience.
2. Data gathering and examination.
3. Chronic disease management.
4. Smoking cessation advice.
5. Reaching a shared management plan.

Domain 1 – Interpersonal skills

Understanding a patient's illness experience

The patient has had a recent scare with the deterioration of his breathing and an asthma attack. How you elicit the patient's story and address his fears and concerns are key skills:

- Start with open questions to allow his story to unfold.
- How does he feel after the hospital visit? What was it like being rushed to hospital? Has it affected how he views his asthma?
- What are his thoughts about having starting smoking again? Does he have any worries about this, e.g. concerns about lung cancer?
- Have recent events impacted on his work or home life, e.g. arguing with his partner?
- What does the patient want from the appointment today? What is his agenda?
- Are there any specific questions he wants answered, e.g. concerns about steroid use?

Domain 2 – Data gathering, technical and assessment skills

Data gathering and examination

Although the consultation needs to be patient-centred, you will have your own agenda too, with specific questions about the history and examination to cover before you feel happy to come to a shared management plan:

- Elicit the history building up to his attendance at hospital. How was he sleeping? Was he wheezy or short of breath? Any chest pain? Was he bringing up phlegm?
- Explore why his asthma has deteriorated over the last few months. Find out about triggers, e.g. smoking, recent chest infections, moving house, new job, pets, new drugs or over-the-counter medications (aspirin, non-steroidal anti-inflammatory drugs [NSAIDs] and β-blockers can all make asthma worse).
- A good screening question if you suspect that his symptoms are related to his occupation is: '*Do your symptoms improve when you are not at work or are on holiday?*'
- Any red flag signs, e.g. weight loss or haemoptysis?
- Given the patient's age, history of smoking and chest tightness, it may be worth quickly asking some cardiac screening questions.

- How have things been since leaving hospital? Has he been using his inhalers and has he taken the tablets prescribed?
- Checking his peak flow could give both you and the patient further reassurance and help establish a baseline reading.
- If his symptoms have resolved and you are happy with his peak flow, further examination is probably not required.

Domain 3 – Clinical management skills

Chronic disease management

This station will test key clinical skills in working in partnership with patients to improve their chronic disease management:

- Assess the patient's understanding of his condition.
- What are his thoughts about managing his condition?
- What is important to him about his asthma – e.g. symptom management?
- Does he understand how his inhalers work? What is his inhaler technique like?
- Does he ever use a peak flow meter to monitor his asthma? Can he use one correctly?
- Are there any barriers to prevent him from coming to regular asthma review appointments?
- Does he understand what to do if his symptoms worsen?
- You could motivate the patient in self-management by empowering him to adjust his medication as appropriate.
- Providing details of self-help support groups and national organizations – e.g. Asthma UK www.asthma.org.uk – would allow him to access peer support and advice.
- You could offer to provide written material to reiterate the points above – e.g. a personalized, written asthma action plan – or use diagrams or models to aid explanations. Check what is in front of you on the desk at this station.

Smoking cessation advice

Smoking cessation advice is a proven cost-effective intervention in primary care, and is all the more important for those with chronic respiratory conditions:

- Where is the patient on the 'cycle of change'? In this case he has relapsed but is contemplating trying to stop again.
- Be extremely positive about any comments he makes about wanting to quit.
- Explore his reasons for stopping smoking previously and emphasize the benefits for his health – use the example of the recent asthma attack to reinforce this point.
- Did he find anything useful last time that helped him stop smoking? His concerns about lung cancer acted as a powerful motivator previously.
- Does he know about the help available now, e.g. nicotine replacement therapy, oral pharmacotherapy and external smoking cessation programmes or nurse-run practice smoking cessation clinics?
- You could reassure him that many people relapse but can still quit again and stay a non-smoker.

Reaching a shared management plan (overlap with domain 1)

The key here is to come to an acceptable management plan that suits this patient's particular life circumstances:

- Try to incorporate the patient's health beliefs into the management plan, e.g. *'Yes, you're right that smoking is making your asthma worse – trying to stop would be the best thing you could do for your health'*.
- Present options that are both realistic and fit with the patient's agenda and priorities. Discussing his thoughts about the way forward is essential. Options might include:
  - Referral to the smoking cessation clinic.
  - Agreeing to review whether to step up or step down his medication after he has attempted to stop smoking (see Knowledge base below).
  - Prescribing a peak flow meter with diary card to allow self-monitoring.
  - Reassurance that nothing suggests a sinister cause of his recent deterioration, e.g. lung cancer. You could offer to let him know when you receive the results of the formal chest x-ray report.
  - Reassurance that steroid tablets for short-term use are safe but best taken in the morning to avoid insomnia.
  - Referral to the nurse for spirometry to assess whether there is any component of chronic obstructive pulmonary disease (COPD) to his condition.
  - Providing information on what to do if his symptoms worsen.
  - Regular follow-up at the nurse-led asthma clinic.

Take-home messages

- It is important to discover and address the patient's health beliefs and behaviours.
- In chronic health conditions such as asthma, patient education, motivation and encouraging self-management are key.
- Safety-netting and appropriate follow-up are essential when dealing with potentially life-threatening conditions.

Tasks

- Re-run the scenario with the patient having recently started work in a bakery alongside the smoking issue. Consider what aspects in the history would point to a diagnosis of occupational asthma.
- Re-run the scenario with the patient attending with an acute exacerbation of asthma using the discharge information regarding PEFR, etc. as your examination findings. (See annex 2 in BTS/SIGN guideline.) How would you manage the patient in your surgery?
- Re-run the scenario with the patient having been successful with smoking cessation and wondering whether the time is right to step down the medication.

Knowledge base

BTS/SIGN British Guideline on the Management of Asthma, January 2012 (www.brit-thoracic.org.uk, www.sign.ac.uk). Reproduced with permission.

Summary of stepwise management in adults

Patients should start treatment at the step most appropriate to the initial severity of their asthma. Check concordance and reconsider diagnosis if response to treatment is unexpectedly poor

MOVE UPTO IMPROVE CONTROL AS NEEDED

MOVE DOWN TO FIND AND MAINTAIN LOWEST CONTROLLING STEP

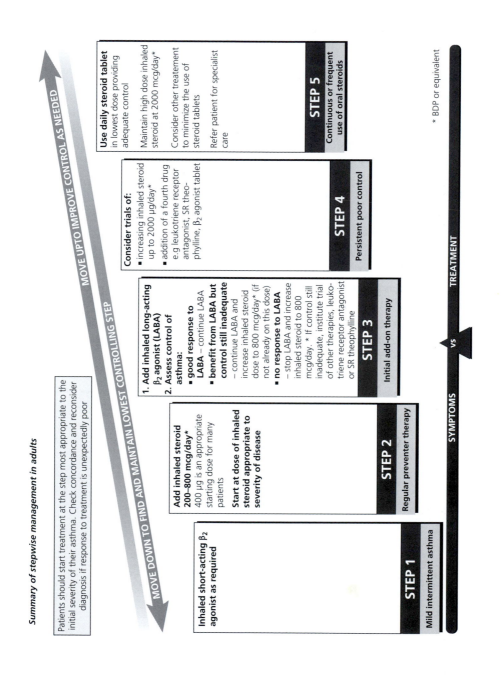

STEP 1

Mild intermittent asthma

Inhaled short-acting β_2 agonist as required

STEP 2

Regular preventer therapy

Add inhaled steroid 200–800 mcg/day*

400 μg is an appropriate starting dose for many patients

Start at dose of inhaled steroid appropriate to severity of disease

---

STEP 3

Initial add-on therapy

1. Add inhaled long-acting β_2 agonist (LABA)

2. Assess control of asthma:
- **good response to LABA** – continue LABA
- **benefit from LABA but control still inadequate** – continue LABA and increase inhaled steroid dose to 800 mcg/day* (if not already on this dose)
- **no response to LABA** – stop LABA and increase inhaled steroid to 800 mcg/day. * If control still inadequate, institute trial of other therapies, leukotriene receptor antagonist or SR theophylline

---

STEP 4

Persistent poor control

Consider trials of:
- increasing inhaled steroid up to 2000 μg/day*
- addition of a fourth drug e.g leukotriene receptor antagonist, SR theophylline, β_2 agonist tablet

---

STEP 5

Continuous or frequent use of oral steroids

Use daily steroid tablet in lowest dose providing adequate control

Maintain high dose inhaled steroid at 2000 mcg/day*

Consider other treatement to minimize the use of steroid tablets

Refer patient for specialist care

SYMPTOMS vs TREATMENT

* BDP or equivalent

1-minute explanations for patients

- Explain the pathophysiology of asthma and the mode of action of the reliever and preventer medication.
- Educate a patient on the correct way to use a metered dose inhaler.
- Explain the mode of action and dosing regimen of Varenicline (Champix®).

Ideas for further revision

In the Clinical Skills Assessment (CSA) there will be a balance of acute and chronic presentations. This station is an example of an acute exacerbation of a chronic condition. Chronic disease management is a key skill expected of GPs, so you should ensure that you feel confident with the management of common chronic conditions seen in primary care, such as diabetes, COPD, asthma and osteoarthritis.

Further reading

Asthma UK free 'Be in Control' pack containing personal asthma action plan for patients www.asthma.org.uk

BTS/SIGN British guideline on the management of asthma, January 2012 www.brit-thoracic.org.uk, www.sign.ac.uk

RCGP curriculum statement 15.8 – Clinical management: respiratory problems www.rcgp.org.uk

Prochaska JO, DiClemente CC. Stages and processes of self-change of smoking: toward an integrative model of change. *Journal of Consulting and Clinical Psychology* 1983; 51: 390–395

STATION 3

Information given to candidates

Mrs Evans is a 44-year-old mother of three children who has asked to see the doctor to talk about her youngest son, Steven, aged 12.

She is attending without her son today.

Steven's records show:

Normal birth and development.

Past medical history – asthma. On beclometasone and salbutamol inhalers.

Sees the asthma nurse regularly – no concerns, good control of asthma.

Other attendances at the GP have been for minor self-limiting illnesses.

Body mass index (BMI) noted to be at 91st centile on last attendance.

As Mrs Evans enters the room she says: 'I'm sorry to bother you, doctor, but I'm worried about Steven's weight.'

- What do you think this station is testing?
- Make notes or discuss your thoughts with a colleague before you read on.

Plan your approach to this station:

Information given to simulated patient

Basic details — You are Janet Evans, a Caucasian 44-year-old mother of three who works part-time in the local baker's.

Appearance and behaviour — You are overweight, well presented and a little anxious.

History

Freely divulged to doctor — You have found out through a friend, whose daughter goes to the same school as your youngest son, Steven, that he is being teased at school about his weight, with other children calling him 'fatty'. Steven has always been a 'heavy' boy but has put on weight over the last year and now appears to weigh more than his 13-year-old brother (although you do not know his exact weight as Steven refuses to go on the scales – he can be a bit sensitive about this). You have tried to get him to play outside more, but his brothers also like to stay in and watch TV or play on the computer, and he has always looked up to, and followed, them. He has even stopped going out with his grandad on the long walks they used to do together.

Divulged to doctor if specifically asked — The family rarely sit down in the evenings to eat together at the kitchen table. Instead the children and your husband eat in front of the television in the front room. You usually eat in the kitchen to get some peace and quiet. In the past you have tried to buy more healthy foods but the children complain that they do not like them. Despite you and your husband working, money is tight, so you often shop at the local budget store, which does not sell fresh fruit or vegetables. You tend to buy the more convenient pre-prepared meals as there is often no time to do a 'proper' meal. Steven is doing fine academically and has always achieved above-average marks at school. Steven has a small group of friends at school, but has seen less of them recently outside school. Steven used to play table tennis regularly at the local youth centre but gradually stopped going last year. Steven has not complained of any aches or pains, and you have not noticed any problems with his mood. He has not wet the bed since he was a toddler. Steven's asthma is well controlled by his inhalers and he regularly attends the asthma nurse clinic at the GP surgery. Apart from his asthma and weight, you have no other health concerns regarding Steven. Lunch at school is provided by the canteen, and you give Steven money for this, although you suspect that he goes to the chip shop instead. Most members of the family are 'heavy', but you only think of Steven as having a problem with his weight. You did not bring Steven today as you first just wanted to discuss things on your own with the doctor.

Ideas, concerns and expectations — You believe that Steven's problems are probably due to eating too much and not doing enough exercise, but you are also worried that his steroid inhaler may be increasing his appetite. You feel a little guilty that if you gave him healthier foods then he would probably not be overweight. You think that taking him to WeightWatchers® might be a way forward, but want to know what the doctor thinks about this – is he too young? You are hoping that the doctor will be able to allay your fears about any serious cause for the weight gain, and to suggest some ways to tackle it.

First words spoken to doctor — 'I'm sorry to bother you, doctor, but I'm worried about Steven's weight.'

Medical history – You have been on anti-depressants for 8 months, but your mood has been good for some time now and you are planning to see the doctor about coming off the medication.

Drug history – You take fluoxetine 20 mg once a day for depression.

Social history – You live with your husband and three children in a council house. You and your husband drink the occasional glass of wine or beer. Neither of you smokes. You work 4 days a week from 10 am to 4 pm at the local baker's and often bring back unsold cakes from work. Your husband works as a roofer. You have a strong marriage. You do all the cooking for the family. Your three sons – Michael 15, James 13 and Steven 12 – get on well together. You drive them the 2 miles to and from school every day. You rarely do physical activities – such as swimming or going on walks – as a family.

Family history – There are no major health problems in the immediate family.

- Having read the information given to the simulated patient, what do you now think this station is testing?
- Make notes or discuss your thoughts with a colleague before you turn the page.

Review your approach to this station:

Tested at this station:

1. Dealing with a third party.
2. History-taking skills.
3. Health promotion and lifestyle advice.
4. Reaching a shared management plan.

Domain 1 – Interpersonal skills

Dealing with a third party

There are always difficulties in conducting a consultation about a patient who is not actually present. In fact, your primary role is often to address the third party's concerns – usually a relative or spouse – rather than dealing with the missing person's 'problem'. Particular issues to consider in this case include:

- Mrs Evans is worried about her son's weight and that he is being called names at school, but you do not know to what extent Steven is particularly bothered by this. You could explore this with her.
- Mrs Evans appears anxious. As you discuss her concerns regarding her son, you need to address, and if possible allay, her anxieties.
- Do you detect any feelings of personal responsibility – or guilt – for Steven's weight gain?
- You could positively reinforce her attendance today by saying how she's made the first step to try to help Steven.

Domain 2 – Data gathering, technical and assessment skills

History-taking skills

You need to try to obtain from Steven's mother as comprehensive a history as you can about his weight gain:

- When did she first notice a problem with his weight?
- How much physical exercise does Steven do? Any sports? Does the family ever do activities together such as swimming or walks?
- What sort of food does Steven eat? Does he eat foods with high sugar and fat content? Does he eat foods rich in salt? How often does he eat fresh fruit and vegetables?
- Where does he eat meals? Do you ever find evidence of Steven eating secretively?
- How is he getting on at school? Has he mentioned the name calling? Any concerns raised by his teachers? Does he have any educational or learning difficulties?
- Does Mrs Evans have any worries about his mood?
- What are her beliefs about eating, activity and weight?
- What is the whole family's lifestyle like? Is Steven's eating behaviour any different from that of his siblings?
- What does your husband think about Steven's weight? What are his views about the family's lifestyle? What are the other children's views?

- Although Steven is not actually present, have you managed to exclude any obvious serious pathology from taking a history from his mother? For example, you could ask about symptoms such as:
  - headache and visual disturbance
  - thirst and polyuria
  - constipation and fatigue
  - early-onset puberty
  - striae and central obesity
  - family history of endocrine disorders.

Domain 3 – Clinical management skills

Health promotion and lifestyle advice

It is important that parents take some responsibility for lifestyle factors in the home, such as diet and eating behaviour, if change is to happen. Points to discuss with Mrs Evans could include:

- How willing are the family to change their lifestyle? Without a positive attitude to change it is unlikely that any modifications will be sustainable.
- Multi component interventions are the most effective at tackling obesity – in other words, it is important to address a whole range of unhealthy behaviours, rather than focus just on, say, diet.
- Increase physical activity – aim for a total of 60 minutes of moderate activity each day. Are there any sports that Steven enjoys but has not done for a while? How might he be encouraged to take these up again?
- Reduce physical inactivity – aim for a limit on the time spent playing computer games or watching TV each day.
- Improve eating behaviour, such as eating together as a family at the table.
- Healthy eating – base meals on starchy foods such as potatoes, rice, pasta and bread and aim for five portions of fruit or vegetables each day. Look to cut down on high-fat and high-sugar foods and drinks.
- Behaviour change strategies, such as goal setting, praise and rewards, and self-monitoring, can all help. Has Mrs Evans tried any of these with Steven?
- What are the barriers to Mrs Evans and her family adopting a healthier lifestyle, e.g. cost, availability of facilities – such as a local leisure centre – and other family members' attitudes? How might these be overcome?
- Adopting a healthier lifestyle could help the whole family in the long term by reducing the risk of heart problems, arthritis and diabetes.

Reaching a shared management plan (overlap with domain 1)

For any plan to be effective you need to make sure that you have taken into account the patient's needs and preferences. In this case you need to think about the whole family, as behavioural change is unlikely to be effective unless it is a joint endeavour. Options you could suggest to Mrs Evans as a way forward include the following:

- Asking Steven to come in to see you for a chat to allow you to conduct a proper assessment, including taking baseline weight and height readings. You need to feel happy that there is no other pathology causing his weight gain.
- Speaking to Steven on his own could reveal his thoughts and feelings about his weight. These need to be incorporated into any management strategy.
- Lifestyle changes for Steven and the whole family in small, manageable and realistic steps might include:
  - Walking to school rather than taking the car – does Mrs Evans think this is feasible?
  - Organizing regular family activities such as going swimming or walks with grandad. Are there any activities the whole family enjoys that involve some physical exertion?
  - Agreeing a limited time spent on the computer each day. Would this be enforceable?
  - Giving Steven and his brothers packed lunches rather than money that can be spent on unhealthy foods. How would the children react?
  - The family agreeing to eat the evening meal together at the kitchen table. What would the family think about this?
  - Mrs Evans not bringing home unsold cakes from her work at the baker's.
- Referral to see a dietitian for further advice and support, such as with meal planning and shopping.
- Self-help or commercial weight-management programmes should be considered only if they are based on a balanced diet, encourage exercise and do not promise excessive weight loss. Mrs Evans may wish to try simple strategies to help improve Steven's lifestyle first.

Knowledge base

National Institute for Health and Clinical Excellence (NICE) (2006 – Updated 2010) CG43 Obesity: the prevention, identification, assessment and management of overweight and obesity in adults and children (Quick Reference Guide 2). London: NICE. Available from www.nice.org.uk/CG043. Reproduced with permission.

Determine degree of overweight or obesity
- Use clinical judgement to decide when to measure weight and height
- Use BMI; relate to UK 1990 BMI charts to give age- and gender-specific information
- Do not use waist circumference routinely; however, it can give information on risk of long-term health problems
- Discuss with the child and family

↓

Consider intervention or assessment
- Consider tailored clinical intervention if BMI at 91st centile or above
- Consider assessing for comorbidities if BMI at 98th centile or above

↓

Assess lifestyle, comorbidities and willingness to change, including:
- presenting symptoms and underlying causes of overweight or obesity
- willingness to change
- risk factors and comorbidities, such as hypertension, hyperinsulinaemia, dyslipidaemia, type 2 diabetes, psychosocial dysfunction, exacerbation of asthma
- psychosocial distress – low self-esteem, bullying
- family history of overweight, obesity and comorbidities
- lifestyle – diet and physical activity
- environment, social and family factors
- growth and pubertal status

↓

Management

Offer multicomponent interventions to encourage:
- increased physical activity
- improved eating behaviour
- healthy eating

Consider referral to a specialist if the child has:
- significant comorbidity or
- complex needs such as learning or educational difficulties

Surgery or appetite-suppressant medication is not recommended for children.

Take-home messages
- Taking a history from a third party can be problematic – encourage the patient to attend for proper assessment.
- Being positive and encouraging change in the whole family is important when trying to help support healthy lifestyle choices for patients.
- Interventions for obesity are more likely to be effective if they are multicomponent, i.e. address diet, eating behaviour and physical activity together.

Tasks

- Re-run the scenario with Mrs Evans reluctantly attending having received a letter from the National Child Measurement Programme highlighting concerns about Steven's weight.
- Re-run the scenario with Mrs Evans enquiring about whether Orlistat can be prescribed for Steven.
- Re-run the scenario changing the family's ethnicity from white European to south Asian and tailoring dietary advice accordingly.

1-minute explanations for patients

- Explain why BMI is used as a measure of obesity.
- Explain the mode of action and prescribing guidance for Orlistat.
- Describe the long-term health impact of being overweight.

Ideas for further revision

The Clinical Skills Assessment (CSA) is unlikely to use child-simulated patients. In order to cover paediatric cases you will therefore be presented with third parties – e.g. a worried parent attending on their own or telephoning for advice. Think about how these scenarios might be set up, e.g. a telephone consultation about a child at home with diarrhoea or parental concerns about self-harm, drug misuse or an eating disorder in their adolescent son/daughter. Next, identify what you would need to know and do in order to score highly at such a station.

Further reading

Department of Health – Why your child's weight matters (leaflet for parents) www.dh.gov.uk/en/Publicationsandstatistics/Publications/PublicationsPolicyAndGuidance/DH_078411

Department of Health – Change4Life for families www.nhs.uk/Change4Life/Pages/change-for-life-families.aspx

NICE clinical guidelines 43: Obesity – Guidance on the prevention, identification, assessment and management of overweight and obesity in adults and children December 2006 (updated 2010) www.nice.org.uk

STATION 4

Information given to candidates

Julie Matcham is a 23-year-old woman who works for a public relations company.

Her notes show that she has been seen twice over the last year with 'mild acne' and has been treated with:

- topical benzoyl peroxide 5% BD prescribed 10 months ago
- oral antibiotics – doxycycline 100 mg OD – commenced 10 days ago.

Her medical history includes irritable bowel syndrome.

For the purpose of the exam, assume that today the patient has mild acne on her face only.

As the patient enters the room she says, 'I was hoping that you could send me to see a skin specialist.'

- What do you think this station is testing?
- Make notes or discuss your thoughts with a colleague before you read on.

Plan your approach to this station:

Information given to simulated patient

Basic details – You are Julie Matcham, a Caucasian 23-year-old recent graduate who works in public relations.

Appearance and behaviour – You appear confident and articulate. You have mild acne on your face only.

History

Freely divulged to doctor – You want to see a skin specialist so you can be prescribed the drug Roaccutane, as you have tried creams and antibiotic tablets for your acne but you think your acne is still bad. From looking on the internet you know that your GP cannot prescribe Roaccutane and that you have to be referred to a specialist first.

Divulged to doctor if specifically asked – You had problems with acne as a teenager but only ever used over-the-counter (OTC) creams. Things flared up about a year ago, soon after you left university and started working, but the acne got better after a month of using the cream prescribed by your GP, so you stopped using it. You saw the GP again 10 days ago as you thought the acne had returned and you were prescribed antibiotic tablets. You know that you are meant to come back in 6–8 weeks for a review, but you feel that things have got worse since you were last seen. When you were back at your parents' home last week you tried using some of your brother's eczema cream, but this just seemed to aggravate your skin. You are otherwise well. Your mood is OK, although you feel less confident at work, due to your skin. Your periods are regular and you have not noticed any excessive facial hair growth. To your knowledge, no family members have polycystic ovary syndrome (PCOS). You split up with your boyfriend last week and are still upset about this. You think that your boyfriend may have left you because of your acne, although he always said he thought your skin was fine.

Ideas, concerns and expectations – A friend mentioned Roaccutane as a possible treatment for acne, although she had only heard of it from a magazine. You are worried about having scars if the acne is not treated properly. You think your acne may have been the reason that you were switched from managing one client to a less high-profile one at work, although your boss explained that the move was due to sickness cover. You are keen to be referred to a specialist to obtain the Roaccutane. However, if the doctor offers you other options for managing your acne and comes across as understanding and competent, then you will consider these.

First words spoken to doctor – 'I was hoping that you could send me to see a skin specialist.'

Medical history – You suffer from irritable bowel syndrome – a feeling of having a bloated abdomen, lower abdominal pain relieved by opening your bowels, and intermittent diarrhoea and constipation – although these symptoms have not bothered you much recently.

Drug history – You have been taking antibiotic tablets – doxycycline 100 mg, one tablet once a day – for 10 days. For several years you have been taking the combined oral contraceptive pill, Microgynon 30. You also take vitamin supplements and occasionally paracetamol for headaches. You are not allergic to any medication.

Social history – You have been working as a new graduate recruit in a public relations firm for about a year. You were living with your boyfriend until recently, when he ended the relationship, and you now share a rented flat with two friends. You have not been going out socializing as much as usual recently as you feel more self-conscious about your skin. You have been wearing more make-up to try to hide your acne.

Family history – Your brother has eczema. There is no family history of serious health problems.

- Having read the information given to the simulated patient, what do you now think this station is testing?
- Make notes or discuss your thoughts with a colleague before you turn the page.

Review your approach to this station:

Tested at this station:

1. Understanding the patient's illness experience.
2. Identifying a hidden agenda.
3. Data gathering.
4. Dealing with a referral request.
5. Reaching a shared management plan.

Domain 1 – Interpersonal skills

Understanding the patient's illness experience

Some dermatological presentations in primary care can appear trivial to doctors, but the GP curriculum stresses the importance of recognizing the social and psychological impact of skin problems on the patient's quality of life:

- You need to explore the patient's perception of the severity of her acne. What makes her think that her skin has got worse recently?
- What effect is her acne having on her work? Any time off work?
- What is the effect on her general functioning? Has her acne affected her confidence levels?
- Has she stopped doing things – such as going out socializing – because of her acne?
- Has anyone else – family, friends or work colleagues – commented on her skin?
- What are her beliefs about the cause of her acne?
- What are her particular worries about the acne?
- What is her general mood like?
- Apart from the referral, was there anything else she wanted to happen as a result of seeing the doctor today?

Identifying a hidden agenda

The GP curriculum says that you need to be aware how cosmetic skin changes can affect patients' interpersonal relationships. This patient will not offer the information about her boyfriend leaving her – and her belief about how her skin was a cause for this – unless you tease this out:

- Why has she decided to attend today?
- Has anything happened recently – any major life events – to prompt her to come back before her routine review appointment scheduled for 6–8 weeks?
- Once you have discovered that she believes her boyfriend left her because of her acne, you need to sensitively explore her reasons for thinking this.
- Has she been focusing on her acne as a way of avoiding confronting the reasons why her relationship ended? Giving her an opportunity to express her thoughts and feelings about what has happened may, in itself, prove therapeutic and help her see her skin problem in perspective.

Domain 2 – Data gathering, technical and assessment skills

Data gathering

Although you are told that the patient has only mild acne, you still need to take a careful history:

- When did her acne first cause her problems? How have things progressed?
- How does she think things are now compared with when she came on her two previous visits 10 days ago and 10 months ago?
- What has she tried for her skin, including OTC and other people's medications? Has anything helped? Does anything make her acne worse?
- Any beliefs about her diet or cleanliness affecting her acne? The GP curriculum says that you should challenge and try to modify any false beliefs around skin problems.
- Is she taking any medication? The progesterone-only pill, topical steroids and phenytoin can all make acne worse.
- Patients may be under the impression that antibiotics may reduce the efficacy of combined oral contraceptives. However, the *British National Formulary* (*BNF*) currently advises that no additional contraceptive precautions are required when combined oral contraceptives are used with antibacterials that do not induce liver enzymes, unless diarrhoea or vomiting occur.
- Does she have flare-ups of her acne that correspond to her periods? Any excessive hair? Any other signs of excess androgens?
- Is she applying topical medication properly, i.e. to all affected areas, not just to spots?
- She thinks that her acne is bad, but objectively it appears only mild. Does she have any other disproportionate concerns about her body, e.g. weight or shape?

Domain 3 – Clinical management skills

Dealing with a referral request

You are required to demonstrate a flexible approach to decision making that incorporates a patient-centred approach. However, the GP curriculum also says that you should recognize the risk of inappropriate referrals:

- Why does she think she needs to see a specialist?
- Has she ever seen a skin specialist before?
- She has tried oral antibiotics for only 10 days and National Institute for Health and Clinical Excellence (NICE) guidelines suggest a minimum of two trials of oral antibiotics before referral to a specialist. Perhaps she could give the current treatment more time?
- She wants to be referred to have isotretinoin (Roaccutane), but does she know that this medication can be prescribed by a GP as a topical preparation? Would she be prepared to consider this?

- She is right that oral isotretinoin (Roaccutane) is prescribed only by a dermatologist, due to the risk of **teratogenicity**. However, does she understand that this is usually considered only after other treatment options have failed or when there are signs of severe acne? Will she accept reassurance from you that her acne is only mild?
- One of the criteria for referral to specialist skin services is psychological distress. Although this patient is upset about breaking up with her boyfriend recently and is worried about her skin affecting her work, she does not appear unduly distressed or psychologically debilitated and there appear to be more appropriate options to try first before considering referral.

Reaching a shared management plan (overlap with domain 1)

This patient wants to be referred, but you could offer her a number of other management options:

- It is always worth giving simple advice such as:
  - do not pick or squeeze spots
  - do not wash excessively and do not use exfoliating agents
  - do not use other people's medication, especially steroid cream.
- How would she feel about trying benzoyl peroxide again? It seemed to help her previously.
- Has she thought about giving the antibiotics longer to work? You could explain that we usually wait 3 months before considering switching to another oral antibiotic and she has been taking the medication for only 10 days.
- What does she think about the option of a topical retinoid, which she has not yet tried? If she does want to proceed then you need to advise her that it can cause skin irritation initially and is contraindicated in pregnancy. She would also need to avoid exposure to ultraviolet light, e.g. apply sunscreen when outdoors and not use sunbeds or sunlamps.
- There is also the option to combine the oral and topical treatments above – what does she think?
- You might be considering co-cyprindiol (Dianette) as an alternative to her combined oral contraceptive pill. However, the *BNF* states that this is licensed for use only in women with severe acne that has not responded to oral antibacterials and for moderately severe hirsutism.
- A referral at this stage would seem inappropriate. You need to be able to explain to the patient in a rational and empathetic manner why this is the case and present her with a number of options, as outlined above.

Knowledge base

References: BNF, NHS Clinical Knowledge Summaries.

Management of acne

Mild to moderate	Topical	Benzoyl peroxide	– available OTC
			– bactericidal
			– consider when inflammatory lesions present
		Antibiotics	– e.g. erythromycin, clindamycin, tetracycline
		Retinoids	– e.g. tretinoin and isotretinoin
			– consider in comedonal acne
		Combined treatments	– combining any two of the three above increases efficacy
		Azelaic acid	– alternative to retinoids and benzoyl peroxide if neither tolerated
Moderate to severe	Oral	In addition to above, consider: Antibiotics	– e.g. first-line: tetracycline, oxytetracycline, doxycycline, lymecycline; second-line: minocycline, erythromycin (latter if tetracycline contraindicated)
			– consider if topical Rx has failed or there is moderate acne on the back or shoulders
			– consider if inflammatory lesions present (risk of scarring)
Severe and unresponsive to above	Oral	In addition to above, consider: Isotretinoin	– prescribed only in secondary care
			– Full blood count (FBC), lipids, liver function tests LFTs and negative pregnancy test before Rx
			– contraception for minimum of 4 weeks before Rx
			– needs careful monitoring as teratogenic
		Trimethoprim	– dermatologist may consider as alternative antibiotic
			– causes a rash in 5% of patients

If a hormonal cause is likely, a combined oral contraceptive or co-cyprindiol (Dianette) may be appropriate. Referral to dermatologist is recommended if:

- poor treatment response
- scarring or pigmentation
- nodulocystic acne
- acne associated with psychological distress.

> **Take-home messages**
> - Always consider why a patient has presented with their problem now. What in particular has triggered their attendance today?
> - When a patient attends with inappropriate referral requests, attempt to offer alternative constructive management options.

Tasks

- Re-run the scenario with a female patient presenting with severe acne.
- Re-run the scenario with a female patient presenting with acne related to PCOS.
- Re-run the scenario with a 40-year-old patient presenting with rosacea.

1-minute explanations for patients

- Describe the natural history and causes of acne.
- Provide self-care advice for patients with mild acne.
- Describe the common triggers for rosacea.

Ideas for further revision

Referral requests could arise in many different Clinical Skills Assessment (CSA) scenarios and can present a challenge to candidates. Look at other scenarios in this book and imagine that a request for a referral has been made. How would you deal with each of these requests in a sensitive yet appropriate manner?

Further reading

Acne Support Group www.stopspots.info/

British Association of Dermatologists – includes patient information leaflets and management guidelines www.bad.org.uk

British National Formulary (*BNF*) – published jointly by BMJ Publishing Group and RPS Publishing, London. Updated every 6 months www.bnf.org

Dermatology Online Atlas – image atlases with diagnoses and differential diagnoses www.dermis.net/dermisroot/en/home/index.htm

NHS Clinical Knowledge Summaries: Acne vulgaris www.cks.nhs.uk/acne_vulgaris

NICE (2010) Referral advice recommendations database www.nice.org.uk

Primary Care Dermatology Society – includes guidelines and recommendations on primary care dermatology www.pcds.org.uk

STATION 5

Information given to candidates

David Foster is a 54-year-old company director with a medical history of hypertension, for which he takes a calcium channel blocker – amlodipine 10 mg OD. His hypertension has been well controlled for several years and the last blood pressure (BP) reading when he saw the nurse 2 days ago was 128/80 mmHg.

His records show that he is a smoker and drinks approximately 42 units of alcohol a week.

When he rang up to request an appointment, Mr Foster was offered the chance to see a nurse practitioner but requested to see a doctor to discuss a 'sensitive' issue.

You know that the patient's wife sees one of your colleagues in the practice and that she is being treated for depression.

When the patient first enters the room and sits down he says, 'It's a bit embarrassing doctor, but I'm finding it difficult to have sex with my wife.'
Assume that physical examination today is normal (including abdomen, genitals, prostate, pulse, BP, peripheral pulses and neurology) and that urinalysis is negative.

- What do you think this station is testing?
- Make notes or discuss your thoughts with a colleague before you read on.

Plan your approach to this station:

Information given to simulated patient

Basic details – You are David Foster, a Caucasian 54-year-old married man and company director.

Appearance and behaviour – You are smartly dressed and articulate, although you are embarrassed and find it hard to discuss the problem for which you have attended today – namely, impotence (also known as erectile dysfunction).

History

Freely divulged to doctor – You are finding it hard to get and maintain an erection to have sex with your wife. This has never been a problem for you in the past. You know that you want to have sex but 'things just don't seem to be working down below'. This is causing arguments between you and your wife.

Divulged to doctor if specifically asked – You had an affair with a female colleague which lasted for 3 months. You ended this relationship 6 months ago as you realized that you had made a terrible mistake and still loved your wife. You have been married for 30 years and have never been unfaithful before. When the affair ended you told your wife what had happened and how you deeply regretted what you had done. Initially you moved out of the house for a month, but since then you have been back at home 'trying to make the relationship work'. You still find your wife sexually attractive. You and your wife have tried to have sex on four or five occasions since you moved back in, but you either cannot get any sort of erection, or your penis gets only semi-erect – not enough for sexual intercourse. You have never used condoms with your wife. You have woken with a full erection on several occasions and you have been able to obtain and maintain an erection for masturbation when you have been alone. When you have masturbated you had no problems ejaculating. Last night on an impulse you went round to the house of the woman you had the affair with and ended up having sex. You deeply regret your actions. You did not have any problems getting or maintaining an erection for intercourse with her. You have not had any discharge from your penis, or any genital irritation. You have never had any sexually transmitted infections (STIs). You are not excessively thirsty. You do not have any genital pain. You have not felt depressed or particularly stressed recently. You have not had any other symptoms such as chest pain, leg pain or numbness.

Ideas, concerns and expectations – You feel guilty about being unfaithful to your wife, especially your actions last night, and also because you think the recent bout of depression that your wife has been suffering from was triggered by telling her about the affair. You are hoping that the doctor can 'check you out' to make sure there are no problems 'down below', although you suspect that the problem is 'in your head'. You used condoms when you had sex with your colleague during the affair and last night, but part of you thinks that you could still have picked up something that you could pass on to your wife. You checked the information leaflet for your BP tablet and saw that sexual dysfunction was listed as a side effect. You have kept taking the medication but you want to ask the doctor about this.

First words spoken to doctor – 'It's a bit embarrassing doctor, but I'm finding it difficult to have sex with my wife.'

Medical history – You were diagnosed with high BP 4 years ago, but your BP has been fine on the tablets. You see the practice nurse every 6 months to get your BP checked.

Drug history – You have been taking a tablet for your BP for more than 3 years: amlodipine 10 mg one tablet once a day. You have not tried any medication to help with your impotence. You are not allergic to any medication.

Social history – You are a director in a successful technology company, which makes circuit boards for mobile phones. You smoke one or two cigars a day. You smoked about 20 cigarettes a day from when you were in your 20s until 10 years ago, when you switched to cigars. You drink a generous glass of whisky most days and a couple of glasses of wine with your evening meal.

Family history – There are no major medical problems in your immediate family.

- Having read the information given to the simulated patient, what do you now think this station is testing?
- Make notes or discuss your thoughts with a colleague before you turn the page.

Review your approach to this station:

Tested at this station:

1. Dealing with a sensitive topic.
2. Data gathering.
3. Taking a sexual history.
4. Physical examination.
5. Reaching a shared management plan.

Domain 1 – Interpersonal skills

Dealing with a sensitive topic

The GP curriculum points out that male genitourinary problems are increasing and men are often embarrassed to present with these conditions. This patient is clearly uncomfortable discussing his erectile dysfunction. You need to try to put the patient at ease by being both empathic and professional:

- Acknowledge his discomfort at having to discuss such a personal matter.
- Explain that such problems are common and that he has made a significant first step in coming to see you today.
- Before you begin taking a history, explain that problems such as his can have physical and psychological causes – and are often a combination of the two – so that he understands your rationale for asking specific questions.
- Take some time to explore his ideas, concerns and expectations. He feels guilty at having the affair and particularly about his actions last night. Taking time now to enquire about these issues should elicit key facts and emotions that will help you identify and address his agenda.
- Discussing sexual matters can be difficult even for healthcare professionals, but if the patient senses any unease or embarrassment on your part then this will compound his discomfort.
- You may have strong personal beliefs about adultery, but you need to remain professional and non-judgemental during the consultation.

Domain 2 – Data gathering, technical and assessment skills

Data gathering

Taking a detailed general history will help you identify the probable cause(s) of his erectile dysfunction:

- How long have the erection problems been going on?
- Any triggers?
- Any previous difficulty getting or maintaining an erection?
- Any previous pelvic surgery?
- Does he have excessive thirst, dysuria, urinary frequency or nocturia?
- Any numbness, weakness, reduced sensation or visual problems?
- Does he suffer from chest pain, pain in his legs when he walks or previous heart or circulation problems?
- Is he able to get an erection if he masturbates? Any problems with ejaculation?

- Does he ever wake up with an erection?
- How has his mood been recently? Is he under particular stress at work?
- How much alcohol does he drink?
- Does he smoke?

Taking a sexual history

Although you will have covered some of the issues around his erectile dysfunction in the general history, it is important not to shy away from taking a specific sexual history for anyone who presents with genital symptoms. In this case, failure to take a detailed sexual history would result in missing a key fact that the patient has managed to have intercourse last night with his colleague, without any erectile dysfunction:

- Signpost the fact that you need to ask some further personal questions about his sexual activity, to help reach a diagnosis. Explain that you ask the same questions of everyone who has these sorts of problems.
- When was the last time he had sex?
- Who was it with? Was it with his wife or with another partner? Was the partner male or female (if this is not immediately obvious from his previous response)?
- Did he use a condom?
- When did he have sex prior to that episode? If this was with a different partner, ask the same set of questions as above.
- Has he had any STIs in the past?
- Any penile discharge?

Physical examination

Patients presenting with erectile dysfunction should be examined to look for hypogonadism (e.g. small or absent testes), secondary sexual characteristics (e.g. gynaecomastia), any signs of penile discharge and structural deformities (e.g. Peyronie's disease). For this station you have been informed that a comprehensive physical examination – including abdomen, genitals, prostate, pulse, BP, peripheral pulses and neurology – together with urinalysis are normal.

Domain 3 – Clinical management skills

Reaching a shared management plan (overlap with domain 1)

As this is a particularly sensitive topic, you need to ensure that any management plan is one that the patient feels comfortable with and has been negotiated to both parties' satisfaction.

- The patient is worried that he may have 'picked something up' through having sex with a different partner. You can reassure him that using condoms greatly reduces the chance of acquiring STIs. But has he considered getting a sexual health check at the local genitourinary medicine (GUM) clinic? This might put his mind at rest regarding having an STI.
- He is concerned that his erectile dysfunction may be related to his BP tablet. Given that he has been taking this medication for 3 years and had not

experienced any impotence prior to his affair, and as he was able to have intercourse last night, you could explain that the tablet is unlikely to be the main cause of his current problems. However, if he wishes to try alternative medication, this would always be an option, although switching drugs could temporarily disturb his otherwise excellent BP control.

- His alcohol intake is excessive – has he considered trying to cut down on his drinking? This could make a significant difference to his erectile problems.
- You can explain that given the history and the normal physical examination there seems to be a large psychological component to his inability to get a full erection with his wife. How does he feel about this suggestion?
- What does he think about couple counselling, such as through RELATE? Would his wife be willing to participate?
- Explain that there are other 'talking therapies' that may help, such as psychosexual counselling.
- Although his problems have a strong psychological component, given his history of smoking, alcohol consumption and high BP, you may wish to discuss doing some routine tests to look at his cholesterol level, blood glucose, liver function tests (LFTs) and kidney function. Other blood tests to exclude a physical component to his erectile dysfunction could include prostate-specific antigen (PSA) and testosterone (morning sample). If the testosterone level is low then prolactin, follicle-stimulating hormone (FSH) and luteinizing hormone (LH) blood tests should also be taken.
- Praise the fact that he cut down from 20 cigarettes a day to one or two cigars. But is he ready to give up completely? This would have a beneficial effect on his general health as well as helping prevent his erectile problems from worsening.
- Explain that there are tablets that can help with erectile dysfunction (see below), but as he does not experience any problems except with his wife, it is probably best first to explore the psychological aspect through counselling. What does he think?
- Arrange to see him in a couple of weeks for follow-up, to discuss the results of any blood tests and to see how things are progressing.

Knowledge base

References – BNF and see Further reading below.

Erectile dysfunction (ED)

Causes – may be multifactorial	Details	Management
Psychogenic	• Generalized (e.g. lack of arousability) or situational (e.g. partner-related) • Usually presents as sudden onset of ED	• Psychosexual counselling • Sensate-focused therapy (stroking only initially: non-genitals, then genitals, then intercourse – therapist gives permission for progression) • Treatments for ED as below may be of benefit

(continued)

Causes – may be multifactorial	Details	Management
Vascular	• Atherosclerosis leading to impaired blood flow to the penis • A detailed cardiovascular history should elicit clues • Usually presents as gradual onset of ED	• Stop smoking if applicable • Assess for other signs of cardiovascular disease (CVD) • Treat modifiable CVD risk factors aggressively (e.g. lifestyle, BP, cholesterol) • Treatments for ED as below may be of benefit
Neurological	• Multiple sclerosis • Parkinson's disease • Stroke • Spinal injury • Cauda equina syndrome • Post surgical (e.g. prostatectomy)	• Treat neurological condition appropriately • Treatments for ED as below may be of benefit
Endocrine	• Diabetes mellitus • Thyroid dysfunction • Hypogonadism • Hyperprolactinaemia	• Urinalysis for glucose and serum glucose • Thyroid function tests (TFTs). Treat any thyroid disease appropriately • Check testosterone levels. Testosterone injections may be indicated • Check prolactin if testosterone levels low
Drug induced	• Excessive alcohol consumption • Anti-hypertensive medication of all classes, most common by diuretics and β-blockers • Anti-depressants • Anti-psychotics • Anti-histamines • Anti-androgens • H2 antagonists	• Reduce alcohol intake • If possible, switch medication to alternatives that do not have ED as a side effect

- First-line pharmacotherapy for erectile dysfunction (once 'curable' causes such as testosterone deficiency have been excluded) includes phosphodiesterase type 5 inhibitors such as sildenafil, tadalafil and vardenafil. These treat erectile dysfunction by increasing blood flow to the penis.
- Such drugs for erectile dysfunction can be prescribed on the National Health Service (NHS) only if the patient has diabetes, multiple sclerosis, Parkinson's disease, poliomyelitis, prostate cancer, severe pelvic injury, spina bifida, spinal cord injury or single gene neurological disease; is on dialysis for renal failure; has had radical pelvic surgery, prostatectomy or kidney transplant; is suffering severe distress (must be prescribed in this case by a specialist centre); or was receiving treatment for erectile dysfunction on the NHS on 14 September 1998.
- Other treatments for erectile dysfunction include sublingual apomorphine, intracavernosal alprostadil injections, intraurethral alprostadil, vacuum devices and penile prostheses.

Tasks

- Re-run the scenario with a 24-year-old patient presenting with premature ejaculation.
- Re-run the scenario with a female patient presenting to discuss her husband's erectile dysfunction.
- Re-run the scenario with the patient having a male partner.

1-minute explanations for patients

- Describe the mechanism of action and side effects of sildenafil.
- Outline the differences between the various pharmacological options for managing erectile dysfunction.
- Provide counselling about lifestyle changes that can help improve erectile dysfunction.

Ideas for further revision

Although the Clinical Skills Assessment (CSA) is primarily an assessment of skills, there will be times when simulated patients put candidates on the spot by asking for a specific piece of factual knowledge. For example, 'How does that drug work, doctor?' or 'But do I have to tell the Driver and Vehicle Licensing Agency (DVLA) about my condition?' Although most candidates sit the Applied Knowledge Test (AKT) some time before the CSA, it is important to maintain, and enhance, your knowledge base as you prepare for the CSA.

Further reading

British National Formulary (BNF) – published jointly by BMJ Publishing Group and RPS Publishing, London. Updated every 6 months www.bnf.org

European Association of Urology – Guidelines on male sexual dysfunction (updated March 2009) www.uroweb.org/gls/pdf/Male%20Sexual%20Dysfunction%202010.pdf

NHS Clinical Knowledge Summaries: erectile dysfunction www.cks.nhs.uk/erectile_dysfunction

Patient UK has clinical summaries specifically designed for doctors, e.g. erectile dysfunction www.patient.co.uk/health/Erectile-Dysfunction-(Impotence).htm

Rabindra G. Erectile dysfunction. *InnovAiT* 2010; 3(1): 44–47

Sexual Dysfunction Association offers information and support for those who suffer from erectile dysfunction, premature or delayed ejaculation, and Peyronie's disease. Online information for patients can be found at www.sda.uk.net

STATION 6

Information given to candidates

> Amy Richards is a 56-year-old woman who has been with the practice for more than 20 years.
>
> She has been taking levothyroxine 75 mcg OD for 8 years. She has regular thyroid function tests (TFTs), which have been stable for several years.
>
> Otherwise she attends the surgery only occasionally with minor self-limiting illnesses.
>
> Her records show that she is often prescribed antibiotics on these occasions.
>
> You note that she normally sees the senior partner when she attends the surgery.

As the patient enters the consultation room she says, 'I need some antibiotics for this ear infection.'
If you perform otoscopy during the consultation, assume that you find no abnormality in either ear.

- What do you think this station is testing?
- Make notes or discuss your thoughts with a colleague before you read on.

Plan your approach to this station:

Information given to simulated patient

Basic details – You are Amy Richards, a Caucasian 56-year-old single woman who works in the local council's finance department.

Appearance and behaviour – You come across as rather demanding.

History

Freely divulged to doctor – Yesterday evening your left ear started aching. This kept you awake much of the night and you have not been able to go into work today because of the pain. You took two paracetamol tablets last night, but thought you would wait to see the doctor before taking any more pills. Your right ear is fine. You want some antibiotics for your 'ear infection'.

Divulged to doctor if specifically asked – You have had a cold, with a runny nose and sore throat for 3 days. Since last night the hearing in your left ear has been a little muffled. You have not noticed any discharge from your ears. Your balance has been fine. You have not had any episodes of dizziness or sensations of spinning. You had a similar 'ear infection' last year for which the senior partner gave you antibiotics (you cannot remember the name of the medication) and this seemed to clear things up within a couple of days.

Ideas, concerns and expectations – You are frustrated at not being able to see the senior partner, who you used to go to school with and usually see for consultations. You think that antibiotics will help your ear problem, as they seemed to do so before. You will find it hard to accept if the doctor says that antibiotics are not immediately indicated. If the senior partner prescribed them before, why is a more junior doctor saying something different today? But you may be persuaded if the doctor treats your concerns with respect and adequately explains your diagnosis and what the best treatment options are.

First words spoken to doctor – 'I need some antibiotics for this ear infection.'

Medical history – You have an under-active thyroid gland and take medication for this daily. You attend the surgery for regular blood tests to check your thyroid hormone levels. These have been fine and your medication dose has remained the same for more than 4 years. Otherwise you come to the surgery occasionally with coughs, colds and minor illnesses, for which you often receive antibiotics.

Drug history – You have been taking levothyroxine 75 µg once a day for 8 years. You are allergic to penicillin – your mother told you that you got a nasty rash and 'swelled up' when you had penicillin as a child.

Social history – You live on your own in a terraced house. You have never smoked and drink a glass or two of wine with your evening meal. You grew up near the GP surgery and have lived and worked in the area ever since. You have an active social life, centred around the local amateur dramatics society.

Family history – Your mother died of breast cancer when she was 88 years old. You have two younger brothers who are fit and well.

- Having read the information given to the simulated patient, what do you now think this station is testing?
- Make notes or discuss your thoughts with a colleague before you turn the page.

Review your approach to this station:

Tested at this station:

1. Dealing with a demanding patient.
2. History-taking skills.
3. Physical examination skills.
4. Management of common medical conditions presenting in primary care.

Domain 1 – Interpersonal skills

Dealing with a demanding patient

Some patients seem to know exactly what they want and during the consultation can come across as demanding. This may invoke negative emotional responses in you that need to be recognized and placed to one side if you are going to manage the consultation in a positive and constructive manner:

- This patient has stated right at the outset what she wants you to do. Acknowledging her request is a good starting point.
- Often patients can appear demanding if they are unhappy about some aspect of their care, e.g. if they have been kept waiting or had problems getting an appointment. In this case the patient wanted to see the senior partner. If you can elicit such issues, e.g. by asking whether there have been any problems with coming to see you today, then you can help defuse any potential conflict in the consultation.
- Why does she believe that she needs antibiotics? How do her previous experiences inform her current demands?
- Exploring her health beliefs around ear problems and antibiotics will help you understand her perspective and help you address any particular concerns she may have.
- What are her worries if she does not have her request met?
- If she insists on demanding a certain course of action, such as antibiotics, you might try explaining the rationale for current best practice, e.g. how we now believe that taking antibiotics for mild, self-limiting infections can increase antibiotic resistance, is unlikely to significantly help recovery, and risks causing unpleasant side effects such as vomiting, diarrhoea and a rash. What does she think about this?
- In this case, the patient has certain expectations in light of her previous consultations. If you refuse to meet her demands today she may simply re-book to see the senior partner who – given his track record – could undermine your actions by prescribing antibiotics to the patient. The scope of the Clinical skills assessment (CSA) includes problem-solving skills and these are meant to include, among other things, being able to adopt a flexible approach to decision making.

Domain 2 – Data gathering, technical and assessment skills

History-taking skills

Although ear pain presenting in primary care is commonly a symptom of a minor, self-limiting illness, it is important to take an adequate history to help rule out more serious diagnoses and guide antibiotic prescribing decisions:

- Are one or both ears affected?
- Are her ears painful?
- Any discharge?
- Has she noticed any problem with her hearing?
- Any sensation of ringing in her ears (tinnitus)?
- Any problems with her balance or sensations of movement, such as spinning?
- Has she had any other symptoms recently, such as a cough or runny nose?
- Has she been feverish or vomited?
- Any previous ear problems?
- What work does she do? Any exposure through work to potential causes of ear problems, e.g. swimming instructor, exposure to loud noise at work?
- Any other pains in her head or neck?
- What medication is she taking? Certain drugs can be ototoxic, such as furosemide and gentamicin.

Physical examination skills

When a patient complains of ear pain or problems with their hearing, a proficient physical examination is required as part of your overall assessment:

- Otoscopy – explain to the patient what will be involved and gain consent before proceeding with the examination:
  - If the patient presents with a problem in one ear, always start by examining the other 'good' ear first.
  - In adults, pulling the pinna backwards and upwards during otoscopy helps straighten out the canal and allows better visualization of the tympanic membrane.
  - Start by examining the pinna and external auditory meatus for debris, discharge or lesions.
  - Examine the external auditory canal for signs of inflammation, swelling, excessive wax or foreign bodies.
  - Can you visualize the tympanic membrane? What colour is it? Any signs of bulging or retraction? Is there an appropriate light reflex? Can you see a fluid level behind the tympanic membrane?
  - If you see a perforation centrally, this is considered safe. However, if the perforation is marginal, it may indicate cholesteatoma and requires referral.
  - Always review patients if you cannot see the tympanic membrane.
- Hearing assessment – in the GP surgery a simple whisper test is adequate for gross hearing assessment. Ask the patient to repeat whispered words with distraction in the other ear by rubbing the tragus.
- Tuning fork tests (512 Hz) – Rinne's and Weber's tests are indicated if the history suggests hearing loss:
  - *Rinne's test* – place the vibrating tuning fork against the bone just behind the patient's ear. Then move the tuning fork beside the external auditory meatus. Ask her which she hears more clearly. If the patient's hearing is normal, or if there is sensorineural hearing loss in that ear, the sound should be heard clearer next to the meatus (air conduction louder than bone conduction). If

she has conductive hearing loss (or severe sensorineural hearing loss) in that ear, she will hear the sound clearer behind the ear.

- *Weber's test* – place the vibrating tuning fork in the middle of the patient's forehead and ask her where she can hear the sound – in the middle or to one side. If she hears the sound to one side, it suggests conductive hearing loss on that side or sensorineural hearing loss on the other side.

Domain 3 – Clinical management skills

Management of common medical conditions presenting in primary care

You need to feel confident about recognizing and managing common ear, nose and throat problems presenting in primary care. The GP curriculum states that you should demonstrate an evidence-based approach to antibiotic prescribing, e.g. in otitis media, to prevent antibiotic resistance:

- You can reassure the patient that on examining her ears there are no signs of any serious infection.
- Does she understand that symptoms of a mild ear infection usually resolve within 3 days without antibiotics?
- Is she prepared to consider 'watchful waiting' as a management option?
- You could reinforce how she has done the right thing in taking painkillers, and advise that self-medication with regular paracetamol and ibuprofen will help her symptoms.
- Delayed antibiotic prescribing – where a prescription is collected by the patient after 3 days if symptoms are not improving or earlier if symptoms worsen – represents another option which may be acceptable to the patient. What does she think about this?
- If you are going to prescribe, remember to ask about allergies – this patient is allergic to penicillin.
- Referral to audiology would be indicated if you had any concerns regarding hearing loss.
- This consultation is also an opportunity for patient education regarding self-management of minor self-limiting illnesses and alternatives to seeing the doctor, such as asking the pharmacist or National Health Service (NHS) Direct for advice.

Knowledge base

References: NHS Clinical Knowledge Summaries, *MeReC Bulletin*.

General	• Ear infections can occur at any age, but are more common in children.

Otitis media	• Inflammation of the middle ear.
	• Acute otitis media (AOM) versus otitis media with effusion (OME) – glue ear:
	  • AOM – often preceded by upper respiratory symptoms (cough, runny nose). Rapid onset. Can present with ear pain, fever, poor sleep and irritability. Signs may include cloudy, bulging or distinctly red or immobile tympanic membrane.
	  • OME – often asymptomatic. Children can present with hearing problems or speech delay, secondary to chronic inflammation and build-up of fluid within middle ear.

(continued)

Acute otitis media (AOM)	• Can be viral or bacterial in origin. • Is usually a self-limiting illness – resolves within 3 days without antibiotics in majority of patients. • Rare complications include mastoiditis, labyrinthitis and meningitis.

Treatment for AOM	• Use of decongestants or antihistamines have insufficient evidence base.
	• Simple analgesics – paracetamol and ibuprofen – can help relieve pain and fever.
	• Antibiotics have been shown to have a modest beneficial effect on the risk of pain after 2 days – 7% absolute risk reduction. But given the risks of side effects and antibiotic resistance they are not recommended routinely for the treatment of AOM.
	• Antibiotics may be indicated if patients:
	  • display systemic features – e.g. vomiting or high fever
	  • experience recurrent infections
	  • have a discharging ear
	  • have bilateral ear infections
	  • are under 2 years old.
	• Where antibiotics are indicated, amoxicillin is considered first-line treatment (child dose: 40 mg/kg TDS – max. 1.5 g daily). Erythromycin can be used for patients allergic to penicillin – as in this scenario – but it is less effective against *Haemophilus influenzae*. Azithromycin and clarithromycin can also be used.
	• Delayed prescribing – prescription to be collected by patient after 3 days if symptoms are not improving or earlier if symptoms worsen – helps reduce antibiotic use and re-attendance rates.

Take-home messages
- Understanding and acknowledging patients' concerns can help defuse potential conflict when they present with demands for treatment.
- The CSA is not designed just to test consultation skills – you must demonstrate proficiency in physical examinations, too.

Tasks
- Re-run the scenario with the patient presenting with a third episode of pharyngitis in 12 months and requesting referral for a tonsillectomy.
- Re-run the scenario with the patient requesting a sick note to say she is unable to work for the next week.
- Re-run the scenario with the patient presenting with headache, vertigo and unilateral conductive hearing loss.

1-minute explanations for patients
- Explain acute otitis media.
- Explain the rationale behind a delayed prescription for antibiotics.
- Explain the diagnosis of a cholesteatoma.

Ideas for further revision
Patient education, including advising on the appropriate use of healthcare resources, is a key part of the GP's role. In your day-to-day practice, do not shy away

from such discussions but instead look to inform patients of the various sources of healthcare advice and support available, which may be more readily accessible, and more appropriate, than booking to see their GP.

Further reading

BMJ topic collections ENT references www.bmj.com/specialties/ear-nose-and-throatotolaryngology

Department for Work and Pensions – A short guide to the benefit system for General Practitioners www.dwp.gov.uk/docs/gp-benefit-guide.pdf

MeReC Bulletin – The management of common infections in primary care. December 2006, 17(3) – section on acute otitis media www.npc.nhs.uk/merec/ infect/commonintro/resources/merec_bulletin_vol17_no3_key_points.pdf

NHS Clinical Knowledge Summaries: otitis media – acute www.cks.nhs.uk/otitis_ media_acute

NICE – Respiratory tract infections – antibiotic prescribing: prescribing of antibiotics for self-limiting respiratory tract infections in adults and children in primary care. CG69 July 2008 http://publications.nice.org.uk/respiratory-tract-infections-antibiotic-prescribing-cg69/introduction

RCGP e-learning course. Self Care for Minor Ailments

http://elearning.rcgp.org.uk/course/view.php?id=80

Information given to candidates

You are a salaried GP, employed by a practice whose senior partner is Dr Mickle. You have worked with Dr Mickle for over a year. He is a competent doctor but under some stress at the moment because of a difficult divorce, which is common knowledge among the practice staff.

Emily Johnson, one of the nurse practitioners, has asked to see you to discuss a patient, Shen Li. She explained in an email that she is concerned with the management of this patient by Dr Mickle.

Mr Li's notes state that he is a 42-year-old builder who had previously been well but then presented complaining of feeling tired for several months. His fasting blood glucose results are recorded as:

7.8 mmol/L – 2 weeks ago
8.4 mmol/L – last week

As she enters the consultation room Emily Johnson says, 'Doctor, you must do something, Dr Mickle is a liability to this practice – he's unsafe as a doctor and extremely rude to colleagues and patients.'

- What do you think this station is testing?
- Make notes or discuss your thoughts with a colleague before you read on.

Plan your approach to this station:

Information given to simulated colleague

Basic details – You are Emily Johnson, a Caucasian 48-year-old nurse practitioner working in a GP surgery. You are qualified to see patients on your own and to manage a range of medical conditions presenting in primary care.

Appearance and behaviour – You are upset and angry at how you have been treated by the senior partner, Dr Mickle. But if the doctor you see today is empathetic and understanding, then you will become more composed.

History

Freely divulged to doctor – You saw a patient, Shen Li, 3 weeks ago with an uncomplicated ear infection. During the consultation he said that he had been feeling tired for several months. You arranged for him to see the practice phlebotomist to have some routine blood tests, including thyroid function tests and a fasting blood glucose test. These were normal apart from a raised glucose – at 7.8 mmol/L. You telephoned the patient and asked him to book to see one of the doctors to discuss the results. The patient asked you on the telephone whether there was anything to worry about and you said that he would need to discuss things with the doctor, but that he probably had diabetes.

Divulged to doctor if specifically asked – You next saw the patient 3 days ago. He told you that, as requested, he had seen Dr Mickle, who had said that it was necessary to repeat the blood glucose test. The patient told you that he had had the second blood test and gone back to see Dr Mickle for the result. (You checked this result on the computer and it was 8.4 mmol/L.) According to the patient, Dr Mickle said his results were nothing to worry about, but that it was important to keep an eye on his blood sugar levels by doing another blood test in 6 months. Mr Li wanted to complain to you about Dr Mickle's manner, saying that Dr Mickle had been dismissive and rude when he (Mr Li) had asked whether he had diabetes. You found this meeting with the patient very difficult as he kept asking why you had said that he had diabetes but Dr Mickle said that he did not. The following day you tried to discuss the matter with Dr Mickle, but Dr Mickle got angry and said that you were not medically qualified and should not be questioning his clinical judgement. Your relationship with Dr Mickle has been a little strained for some time, ever since you felt that he had blocked your suggestions for developing the minor illness service at the surgery last year. You do not know about any other incidents with patients where Dr Mickle's management has given any cause for concern. Dr Mickle seems to have been rather short-tempered this last month and has had several days off for illness recently, which is quite unlike him. You told the patient that you would discuss the matter with Dr Mickle and see the patient again to try to answer his questions about his diagnosis.

Ideas, concerns and expectations – You think Dr Mickle has missed the diagnosis of diabetes mellitus in the patient Shen Li. You do not understand why he would have made this error. You do not really think that he is 'unsafe as a doctor', but you are upset about how he has behaved towards you. You did not like being made to look stupid and you are worried that relations with Dr Mickle – who is the senior partner and your employer – have deteriorated further. You want to try to resolve the situation and hope that the doctor you are seeing today will be able to somehow 'sort out this mess'. You would be happy to attend a meeting with Dr Mickle if someone else was there to give you support.

You would also be happy if the doctor wants to discuss things first with Dr Mickle on his own, or to seek advice from others on how best to proceed.

First words spoken to doctor – 'Doctor, you must do something, Dr Mickle is a liability to this practice – he's unsafe as a doctor and extremely rude to colleagues and patients.'

Medical history – You are fit and well and have never suffered from any significant medical problems.

Drug history – You do not take any regular medication.

Social history – You work full-time at the GP surgery and live with your husband and teenage son.

Family history – There are no significant medical problems in your immediate family.

- Having read the information given to the simulated patient, what do you now think this station is testing?
- Make notes or discuss your thoughts with a colleague before you turn the page.

Review your approach to this station:

Tested at this station:

1. Providing support to a colleague.
2. Gathering information in relation to a complaint.
3. Dealing with a complaint about a colleague.
4. Understanding patient safety issues.

Domain 1 – Interpersonal skills

Providing support to a colleague

One of your colleagues is visibly distressed at events at work. She has chosen to speak to you about this matter and you need to be understanding and supportive in your response:

- Allow her to freely express her thoughts about what has happened. Use active listening skills to demonstrate your attentiveness, together with open questions to encourage her to fully disclose her perspective on events.
- Empathize with her situation and the stressful meetings she has had with both the patient and Dr Mickle.
- Ask her what she was hoping you could do to help.
- If she wants to discuss the matter again with Dr Mickle but would like someone else there for support, you could offer to arrange the meeting and be present.

Domain 2 – Data gathering, technical and assessment skills

Gathering information in relation to a complaint

After you have given the nurse practitioner an opportunity to tell her story, it is important to try to ascertain her precise account of events. More specific closed questions may help you in this regard:

- Can she tell you when she first thought there was a problem?
- Can she describe exactly what happened at each meeting with the patient? When did these take place?
- When she tried to discuss the matter with Dr Mickle, what happened?
- What makes her say that Dr Mickle is 'unsafe as a doctor'? Have there been any other incidents involving Dr Mickle that she would like to discuss?
- She says that the patient told her that Dr Mickle was rude to him. Can she say more about this? Has the patient made a formal complaint?
- Does she know who took the blood samples? Were they definitely fasting samples?
- What arrangements have been made with the patient for follow-up?

Domain 3 – Clinical management skills

Dealing with a complaint about a colleague

One of the members of your clinical team has made a complaint about another doctor you both work alongside. You need to take this seriously and act appropriately:

- As the GP curriculum makes clear, all health professionals are expected to adhere to ethical principles which are the framework for professional codes of conduct (see knowledge base and further reading below).
- These codes outline minimum standards of practice and limits to behaviour.
- The allegations put to you are that one of your medical colleagues:
  - incorrectly reassured a patient that he did not have diabetes
  - was rude and dismissive when the matter was raised with him by a fellow health professional
  - was rude to the patient involved.
- According to the nurse practitioner, Dr Mickle's recent behaviour is out of character for him. There is also the suggestion that his health may be suffering – he has taken several days off sick recently, which is quite unlike him. His short temper and time off work could be related to his divorce. Although his divorce is common knowledge among practice staff it is probably best not to mention this directly, although you could agree that he does appear to have been rather stressed recently.
- You cannot fully understand the situation without discussing the matter with Dr Mickle. For example, it may be that the blood tests were not in fact fasting samples and this is why Dr Mickle has reassured the patient that he does not have diabetes. However, even if this turns out to be the case, there are still questions over Dr Mickle's professional behaviour towards his colleague and the patient.

Understanding patient safety issues

When a concern is raised about a colleague, your first priority must be to ascertain whether patients have been, or are likely to be, put at risk:

- You could make clear to the nurse practitioner that if a mistake has been made, you would be happy to explain this to the patient, apologize, and describe what steps will be taken to reduce the chance of this happening again. However, first you need to speak to Dr Mickle, both to gather more information and to offer him some support.
- As the Royal College of General Practice and the British Medical Association make clear (see Knowledge base below), when relationships within the healthcare team break down, patient care usually suffers. Therefore, from a patient safety perspective it is important to try to resolve the dispute between the nurse practitioner and Dr Mickle.
- Reflective practice around patient safety issues is a key opportunity for staff and organizations to learn about, and improve, patient care. So it is important to have an open and constructive approach to discussing incidents where concerns have been raised about patient safety. One way forward would therefore be to propose a practice meeting to discuss the criteria for diagnosing diabetes.
- In summary, your options include:
  - offering to arrange a meeting with Dr Mickle on his own
  - offering to arrange a meeting with Dr Mickle and the nurse practitioner
  - offering to see the patient, once you have ascertained further information about events
  - organizing a practice meeting reviewing criteria for diabetes diagnosis and perhaps suggesting a practice policy or guideline.

Knowledge base

Professional and ethical issues

References: GMC guidance, RCGP and BMA guidance – see Further reading below.

GMC Good Medical Practice 2009 update	Good doctors (para 1)	• Good doctors make the care of their patients their first concern: they are competent, keep their knowledge up to date, establish and maintain good relationships with patients and colleagues, are honest and trustworthy, and act with integrity.
	Working in teams (para 41)	• When working in a team, you should act as a positive role model and try to motivate and inspire your colleagues. You must respect the skills and contributions of your colleagues.
	Conduct and performance of colleagues (para 43)	• You must protect patients from risk of harm posed by another colleague's conduct, performance or health. The safety of patients must come first at all times. If you have concerns that a colleague may not be fit to practise, you must take appropriate steps without delay, so that the concerns are investigated and patients protected where necessary.
	Respect for colleagues (para 46)	• You must treat your colleagues fairly and with respect [...] You should challenge colleagues if their behaviour does not comply with this guidance.
RCGP and BMA Good Medical Practice for General Practitioners 2008	Working in teams (pp. 36–38)	• Good team working includes respecting colleagues both personally and professionally. • When relationships within the team break down, patient care usually suffers. Therefore, ensuring good communication within your team is an important part of being a good GP.
	Health (pp. 53–54)	The exemplary GP: • is aware when a colleague's performance, conduct or health might be putting patients at risk • quickly and discreetly ascertains the facts of the case, takes advice from colleagues and, if appropriate, refers the colleague to the responsible officer in the primary care organization for local investigation • provides positive support to colleagues who are ill, who have made mistakes or whose performance gives cause for concern as part of agreed procedures • realizes when his or her own performance is unsafe, e.g. through illness, and seeks and follows advice from a suitable colleague, taking any action required to reduce patient risk.

Diabetes mellitus diagnosis

References: WHO 1999, 2006 and 2011 – see Further reading below.

Diagnosis	Findings

Diabetes mellitus	• Symptomatic
	  • with 1 random blood glucose ≥11.1 mmol/L
	  • with 1 fasting blood glucose ≥7.0 mmol/L

	• Asymptomatic
	  • with 2 random blood glucose results on different days ≥11.1 mmol/L
	  • with 2 fasting blood glucose results on different days ≥7.0 mmol/L

	• Glucose tolerance test – give 75 mg glucose to fasting patient, take sample after 2 hours • blood glucose ≥11.1 mmol/L
	• Glycated haemoglobin (HbA1c) ≥6.5%
Impaired fasting glycaemia	• Fasting blood glucose ≥6.1 mmol/L and <7.0 mmol/L • And (if measured) blood glucose <7.8 mmol/L 2 hours post glucose load in glucose tolerance test
Impaired glucose tolerance	• Glucose tolerance test • blood glucose ≥7.8 mmol/L and <11.1 mmol/L 2 hours post glucose load

> **Take-home messages**
> - You need to be aware of the professional ethical guidelines which are central to your practice as a GP.
> - When patients or colleagues come to you with a complaint, you can be supportive and understanding without having to make an immediate judgement as to the merit of the complaint.
> - Patient safety must always take priority.

Tasks

- Try re-running the scenario with the simulated colleague replaced by the simulated patient (Shen Li). How might you respond to the patient's questioning regarding whether he has diabetes or not? What would you say if he criticizes your healthcare colleagues?
- Try re-running the scenario with the nurse practitioner alleging that Dr Mickle is turning up to work smelling of alcohol. What sources of support are available for doctors with health or addiction problems?
- For international candidates (e.g. those undertaking the MRCGP[INT]) who may be working in a single-handed practice without a nurse practitioner, try re-running the scenario with the patient complaining about a locum who was in charge while you were away. The patient wants to complain as he's found out from a relative who is a doctor that his blood tests show that he has diabetes.

1-minute explanations for patients

- Explain how you diagnose diabetes mellitus.
- Explain what diabetes mellitus is.
- Explain your practice's complaints procedure.

Ideas for further revision

This station is primarily looking at relationships with colleagues and patient safety issues. However, it is important to be familiar with the diagnostic criteria for diabetes mellitus to help in your response. Other Clinical Skills Assesment (CSA) stations may focus on data interpretation in more detail and you should feel comfortable interpreting blood test results, child growth charts, cervical smear reports, spirometry graphs, imaging reports, electrocardiographs and other clinical test results that are commonly seen in general practice.

Further reading

Association of British Clinical Diabetologists www.diabetologists-abcd.org.uk

General Medical Council. Good Medical Practice. London: GMC, updated 2009 www.gmc-uk.org/static/documents/content/GMP_0910.pdf

National Patient Safety Agency www.npsa.nhs.uk

RCGP curriculum statements – Personal and professional responsibilities: 3.2 Patient safety; 3.3 Clinical ethics and values-based practice www.rcgp-curriculum.org.uk/curriculum_documents/gp_curriculum_statements.aspx

Royal College of General Practitioners and General Practitioners Committee of the BMA. Good Medical Practice for General Practitioners. London: Royal College of General Practitioners, 2008 www.rcgp.org.uk/pdf/PDS_Good_Medical_Practice_for_GPs_July_2008.pdf

World Health Organization. Use of glycated haemoglobin (HbA1c) in the diagnosis of diabetes mellitus: abbreviated report of a WHO consultation. Geneva 2011 www.who.int/diabetes/publications/report-hba1c_2011.pdf

World Health Organization. Definition, diagnosis and classification of diabetes mellitus and its complications 1999 www.staff.ncl.ac.uk/philip.home/who_dmc.htm

World Health Organization and International Diabetes Federation. Definition and diagnosis of diabetes mellitus and intermediate hyperglycaemia. Geneva 2006 http://whqlibdoc.who.int/publications/2006/9241594934_eng.pdf

Information given to candidates

Wesley Anderson is a 58-year-old black British man, whose parents come from the Caribbean, who rarely attends the surgery.

He attended 1 month ago with a sprained right ankle, injured while playing football, which resolved with ibuprofen.

He had his blood pressure (BP) routinely checked at that time and it was 150/94 mmHg. This was repeated later in the same consultation and was again 150/94 mmHg in both arms. Cardiovascular examination and fundoscopy were otherwise normal. Urine dip-stick was normal. Various blood tests, a further urine test and an electrocardiogram (ECG) were requested. Ambulatory blood pressure monitoring (ABPM) was arranged. He was given lifestyle advice.

He has returned today for the results of the various investigations

Full blood count (FBC) – normal	Height – 180 cm
Urea and electrolytes (U & Es) – normal	Weight – 100.4 kg
Estimated glomerular filtration rate (eGFR) – normal	Body mass index (BMI) – 31 kg/m²
Liver function tests (LFTs) – normal	
Glucose – normal	
Total cholesterol – 6.0 mmol/L	ECG – sinus rhythm; no abnormality seen;
High-density lipoprotein (HDL) – 1.0 mmol/L	heart rate 72
Urine albumin: creatinine ratio (ACR) <2.0	
ABPM – average daytime reading of 146/92 mmHg	

As the patient enters the room he says, 'I've come to get the results of all the tests you people arranged.'
On the desk in front of you are cardiovascular risk prediction charts (reproduced in the back of the British National Formulary (BNF)).

- What do you think this station is testing?
- Make notes or discuss your thoughts with a colleague before you read on.

Plan your approach to this station:

Information given to simulated patient

Basic details – You are Wesley Anderson, a 58-year-old black British man who was born and brought up in the UK but whose parents came from the Caribbean.

Appearance and behaviour – You are well presented and somewhat overweight.

History

Freely divulged to doctor – You came to see the doctor 1 month ago after injuring your right ankle and a routine blood pressure check found that it was up a little. The doctor arranged some blood tests, a urine test, a heart recording (ECG) and a blood pressure machine that you had to wear for 24 hours while it took various readings. You also had a long discussion about changes you could make to your diet and lifestyle to try to get your blood pressure down. The doctor also 'nagged' you about stopping smoking. You have come back today for the results of all these tests. You feel 'a bit of a fraud' as you feel so well.

Divulged to doctor if specifically asked – Over the last month you have tried to eat a healthier diet but it has been difficult. You know that you are overweight but this does not really bother you. You think of yourself as fairly fit for your age. You still play football with your sons and friends in the park on Sundays. You have never had any chest pains, shortness of breath, palpitations, headaches or any other symptoms that have worried you. You drink five or six cups of coffee most days. You know that you should quit smoking but you just don't feel ready to do this at the moment.

Ideas, concerns and expectations – Although today you are seeing a different GP about your blood pressure, you are not bothered by this – the previous doctor seemed very thorough – and you understand that it is not always possible to see the same doctor. You are a little confused about why the doctors seem so interested in your blood pressure when you feel absolutely fine and have not had any symptoms. Last time the doctor mentioned that you might need to take tablets for the rest of your life, which bothers you as you have always thought of yourself as a healthy individual and not someone who takes tablets. You were not sure what all the blood tests and other tests were for and you are a little worried that there may be something else that the doctors have not mentioned, to warrant all the tests. You bought a relaxation tape as you thought this might help your blood pressure and you want to ask the doctor about this.

First words spoken to doctor – 'I've come to get the results of all the tests you people arranged.'

Medical history – You rarely come to see the doctor. When you were with your previous GP surgery, you suffered from gout in your left big toe on two occasions
4 years ago but have been fine since. You sprained your right ankle playing football
2 weeks ago and only booked to come to see the GP at your partner's insistence as she thought you might have broken something. The ankle problem cleared up quickly with anti-inflammatory painkillers.

Drug history – You were prescribed medication to help prevent further gout attacks when you were registered at your previous practice, but you decided not to take it. You do not take any regular medication. You are not allergic to any drugs.

Social history – You live with your partner and two adult sons in a semi-detached house. You have run your own business – selling kitchen units – for 30 years. You drive a small van for work. You have smoked 20 cigarettes a day since you were 15 years old. You know that you drink a little too much – you often have four pints of lager on Friday and Saturday nights in the local pub, and one or two cans of lager most week nights at home after work.

Family history – Your father died of a heart attack when he was 72. Your mother had high blood pressure in her 70s but did not need any tablets for it. She died of breast cancer aged 76. Your older brother has had high blood pressure for the last 5 years. He is now 65 years old. He takes a couple of tablets every day but is otherwise well.

- Having read the information given to the simulated patient, what do you now think this station is testing?
- Make notes or discuss your thoughts with a colleague before you turn the page.

Review your approach to this station:

Tested at this station:

1. Data gathering.
2. Data interpretation.
3. Explanation of diagnosis.
4. Management of common medical conditions presenting in primary care.

Domain 1 – Data gathering, technical and assessment skills

Data gathering

This patient has been found to have raised BP confirmed by ABPM. Data gathering at this station should include appropriate patient-centred history taking and review of the results of his various investigations:

- History – you should elicit most of the following:
  - Does he smoke?
  - Any family history of heart attacks, heart problems, high BP or strokes?
  - Any chest pain, palpitations or shortness of breath?
  - Does he ever wake up at night gasping for breath? How many pillows does he use at night? Do his ankles swell up?
  - Any problems with pains in his legs when he walks?
  - Any headaches?
  - You already know that he is not diabetic from the blood glucose result.
  - Any family history of high cholesterol?
  - Any other medical problems in the past?
  - Does he take any medication?
- BP readings – ABPM readings show a daytime average of ≥135/85 mmHg (but <150/95 mmHg). Therefore he meets the criteria for stage 1 hypertension (see Knowledge base below).
- Other tests – investigations to look for signs of end organ damage (from blood tests, urine ACR and ECG) or diabetes. Total cholesterol:HDL ratio is 6. BMI is 31 kg/m^2.

Data interpretation

In addition to the results of the patient's recent blood tests, ECG, urine ACR and ABPM readings, you have access to cardiovascular risk prediction charts (also found in the back of the *BNF*). You need to be able to demonstrate that you can interpret these data in light of current best practice guidelines to help inform management options:

- Given his age, raised BP and cholesterol ratio, you should calculate his cardiovascular disease (CVD) risk to see whether he needs to be on appropriate treatment.
- CVD risk is defined as non-fatal myocardial infarction (MI) and stroke, coronary and stroke death and new angina pectoris.
- Note that when deciding whether to use the 'Non-smoker' or 'Smoker' risk prediction charts, it is recommended that you should assess those who have

given up smoking within 5 years using the 'Smoker' charts. In this case the patient is still smoking.

- CVD risk is underestimated by the charts for those with a family history of premature CVD – namely, female first-degree relative aged <65 years or male <55 years. However, this patient's father was 72 years old when he had his heart attack.
- Select the appropriate risk prediction chart – namely 'Non-diabetic men' and 'Smoker' and 'Age 50–59'.
- From the blood test results you know that the total cholesterol (TC): HDL ratio is 6.0: 1.0 = 6. If you plot where the x axis for TC : HDL of six intersects with a systolic BP of 146 mmHg you can see that this is clearly within the CVD risk >20% over the next 10 years. Hence this patient is at significant CVD risk.
- The risk prediction charts may underestimate CVD risk in some ethnic minorities. In patients from the Indian sub-continent it is recommended to multiply the calculated risk by 1.5 to obtain a more realistic value. This patient is black British with parents from the Caribbean. There are tools such as the ETHRISK calculator which adjusts the CVD risk for certain ethnic groups (see Further reading below).

Domain 2 – Interpersonal skills

Explanation of diagnosis

Explaining to patients what you think is wrong with them in terms that they can readily understand and which incorporate their health beliefs is a key communication skill:

- You are the second health professional this patient has seen about his BP. What did the other doctor explain about high BP?
- What are his health beliefs about BP? Are any family members or friends having treatment for BP? Has he discussed the matter with them?
- Does he have any concerns about all this interest in his BP? What was he expecting would happen at today's appointment?
- Does he know why we are interested in raised BP, even when someone does not have any symptoms? You need to explain our understanding that over time high BP can damage blood vessels and put a strain on the heart.
- Does he understand why the other doctor ordered the various tests? You could explain how the tests look at different things – to confirm that his BP is high, whether there are any problems with his kidneys or heart, whether he has diabetes, and whether his cholesterol is raised.
- Communicating risk – you can explain how we calculate the patient's risk of developing CVD. If someone scores ≥20% – in other words a 2 out of 10 chance or more – of developing CVD in the next 10 years then you can make clear that we usually advise starting medication.
- You can explain that treatment may include drugs to lower BP and a statin drug to lower cholesterol. But lifestyle factors such as stopping smoking, diet and exercise are also very important (see below).

- You can use the risk assessment process to aid discussion with the patient and potentially encourage concordance, e.g. showing him the charts and demonstrating how getting his cholesterol and BP down can reduce his risk.
- It is worth asking how the patient feels about having high BP. His self-image as a fit, healthy individual was challenged by the previous doctor's mention of having to take medication long term.
- This patient wants advice on the use of relaxation tapes. He is already starting to think about taking some responsibility for his BP management and you should positively reinforce this behaviour. You can tell him that relaxation techniques may lead to modest reductions in BP.

Domain 3 – Clinical management skills

Management of common medical conditions presenting in primary care

Management of the risk factors for cardiovascular problems is a key aspect of health promotion activity in primary care. Hypertension is one modifiable risk factor that all GPs should feel confident in treating:

- Lifestyle advice is a key element in controlling BP whether or not patients require anti-hypertensive medication. You should positively reinforce the fact that he is physically active, and discuss how he might try to address his alcohol intake and weight. Dietary advice to help reduce BP should include cutting down on salt and discouraging excessive caffeine consumption. Most importantly, the goal of trying to stop smoking should be discussed.
- The patient meets the threshold to be offered drug therapy for his hypertension (stage 1 hypertension). According to National Institute for Health and Clinical Excellence (NICE) guidelines, calcium channel blockers would be a first-line option given his profile (see Knowledge base below).
- If you are going to write a prescription for him today, you might consider starting amlodipine 5 mg OD. Remember to discuss with him side effects, such as abdominal pain, nausea, palpitations and swollen ankles. Is he happy to take this medication?
- What does he think about cholesterol-lowering tablets? Does he understand how it can help reduce his CVD risk? Simvastatin 40 mg nocte would be one option. However, another option is to see if he can try to address other modifiable CVD risk factors such as smoking, weight, alcohol consumption and BP first.
- Do not forget to check allergy status before prescribing any drugs – this patient has no known allergies.
- He did not take his gout prophylaxis medication previously, when prescribed. You need to understand his reasons for this as his past behaviour may be relevant to future concordance in relation to his anti-hypertensive tablets.
- The GP curriculum notes that many patients do not take their preventative cardiovascular medication and that you need to respect patient autonomy when reaching a management plan. Is he really planning to take his new medication and does he have any further questions about the tablets?
- It might be prudent to check his urate levels, given his history of gout.
- Ask him to see you again in 4 weeks for a review, or sooner if he has any concerns.

Knowledge base

References: NICE Guidelines 2011 and 2008, *BNF*, DVLA 2011.

Hypertension	• Stage 1 hypertension: clinic BP ≥140/90 mmHg and ABPM daytime average or home BP monitoring average ≥135/85 mmHg.
	• Stage 2 hypertension: clinic BP ≥160/100 mmHg and ABPM daytime average or home BP monitoring average ≥150/95 mmHg.
	• Severe hypertension: clinic BP ≥180/110 mmHg.
Lifestyle advice	• Offer lifestyle advice initially and then periodically for those being assessed or treated for hypertension.

Anti-hypertensive drug therapy	• Offer drug treatment if:
	  • stage 1 hypertension, aged under 80 years, with: target organ damage, established CVD, renal disease, diabetes or CVD risk ≥20% over 10 years
	  • stage 2 hypertension of any age.

Treatment targets	• Clinic readings <140/90 mmHg in people aged under 80 years. • Clinic readings <150/90 mmHg in people aged 80 years and over.
Cholesterol	• Statins – used for primary prevention to reduce CVD risk in those aged over 40 years with ↑BP who have CVD risk ≥20% over 10 years.
Elderly patients	• If they meet the criteria for drug treatment, offer the same anti-hypertensive drug treatment to patients aged 80 years and over as you would to those aged 55–80 years, bearing in mind comorbidities and drug interactions.
Secondary causes of ↑BP	• Kidney disease (e.g. renal artery stenosis). • Cushing's syndrome. • Conn's syndrome. • Hyperparathyroidism. • Acromegaly. • Phaeochromocytoma. • Coarctation of aorta.
Driver and Vehicle Licensing Agency	• Group 1 drivers – can continue driving and not required to inform DVLA unless treatment causes unacceptable side effects. • Group 2 drivers – stop driving and notify DVLA if resting systolic pressure ≥180 mmHg or resting diastolic pressure ≥100 mmHg.
Continuing care	• Annual review with patients to monitor BP, discuss lifestyle, provide support, assess medication use and side effects.

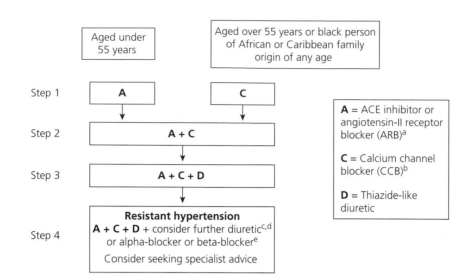

^a Choose a low-cost angiotensin-receptor blocker.

^b A calcium channel blocker (CCB) is preferred but consider a thiazide-like diuretic if a CCB is not tolerated or the person has oedema, evidence of heart failure or high risk of heart failure.

^c Consider a low-dose spironolactone^d or higher doses of a thiazide-like diuretic.

^d At the time of publication (August 2011), Spironolactone did not have a UK marketing authorization for this indication. Informed consent should be obtained and documented.

^e Consider an α-blocker or β-blocker if further diuretic therapy is not tolerated, or is contraindicated or ineffective.

Take-home messages

- Data interpretation is a key skill that can be assessed in the CSA.
- Explain diagnoses to patients in terms they can understand.
- Lifestyle advice is a fundamental element in the management of hypertension.

Tasks

- Try re-running the scenario with this patient aged 36 years, then again with the patient aged 82 years. How might your data gathering and management change in each case?
- Try re-running the scenario with a patient from the Indian sub-continent across these different age ranges. How might your data gathering and management change in each case?
- Try re-running the scenario with the patient returning for his review at 1 month. What clinic target BP are you aiming for? What would you do if he was having unpleasant side effects from the amlodipine?

1-minute explanations for patients

- Explain dietary changes to help reduce cholesterol.
- Explain how amlodipine works.
- Explain how statins work.

Ideas for further revision

Explaining new diagnoses to patients is a common occurrence in primary care. Practise trying to explain diagnoses such as osteoarthritis, chronic obstructive pulmonary disease, asthma, diabetes and thyroid disease in simple, accurate, jargon-free terms.

Further reading

British Hypertension Society www.bhsoc.org/default.stm

Cardiovascular Risk Prediction Charts; at back of the *BNF*. Published jointly by BMJ Publishing Group and RPS Publishing, London. Updated every 6 months www.bnf.org

DVLA Swansea. For Medical Practitioners: At a glance guide to the current medical standards of fitness to drive. August 2011 www.dvla.gov.uk/medical/ataglance.aspx

ETHRISK – A modified Framingham CHD and CVD risk calculator for British black and minority ethnic groups www.epi.bris.ac.uk/CVDethrisk

NICE guidelines – Hypertension: Clinical management of primary hypertension in adults. Clinical guidelines 127 (update of NICE clinical guidelines 34) August 2011. Quick reference guide available at: www.nice.org.uk/nicemedia/live/13561/56015/56015.pdf

NICE guidelines – Lipid modification. Clinical guidelines 67. May 2008 (reissued March 2010). Quick reference guide available at: www.nice.org.uk/nicemedia/live/11982/40675/40675.pdf

RCGP curriculum statement 15.1 – Clinical management: cardiovascular problems www.rcgp.org.uk

STATION 9

Information given to candidates

Mavis O'Brien is a 74-year-old patient and mother of one of the practice nurses.

Her medical history includes a myocardial infarction (MI) 10 years ago. She has not had angina pains since the MI.

She is prescribed the following medication:

Aspirin 75 mg OD
Bisoprolol 5 mg OD
Ramipril 2.5 mg OD
Simvastatin 40 mg nocte

At the last consultation 6 months ago, the patient was very upset over the death of Edna, her best friend.

The first thing the patient says as she enters the consultation room is, 'I've been getting ever so dizzy, doctor, over the last few months, I wonder if it's to do with my nerves. I want you to sort me out.'

- What do you think this station is testing?
- Make notes or discuss your thoughts with a colleague before you read on.

Plan your approach to this station:

Information given to simulated patient

Basic details – You are Mavis O'Brien, a Caucasian 74-year-old retired schoolteacher and widow.

Appearance and behaviour – You are anxious and fidgety, and talk rather fast. But if you feel the doctor is kind and understanding then you will begin to relax a little and slow down. During the consultation you repeatedly ask the doctor if he or she can 'sort things out' for you.

History

Freely divulged to doctor – You started having dizzy spells 5 or 6 months ago. They can last from a few seconds to several minutes. Your daughter thought that you should come to see the doctor as she is worried about your symptoms, although you have never blacked out or fallen during these episodes. You miss your friend and companion Edna terribly since she died 6 months ago, and you think that the dizziness may be due to her death affecting your 'nerves'.

Divulged to doctor if specifically asked – You find it hard to describe exactly what the dizziness feels like. The best description you can give is that you feel a little lightheaded. Sometimes you get several episodes of dizziness in one day, then nothing for over a week. There does not seem to be any pattern to when they come on – for instance, you have not noticed things being worse after you stand up, or if you move your head suddenly. You do seem to get more anxious these days and when you are dizzy you sometimes notice that you are breathing faster. Your ears have been fine. You have not experienced any chest pain, palpitations, weakness or odd sensations in your limbs. You do not feel sick or particularly unsteady on your feet when the dizziness comes on. You have not noticed any problem with your eyesight. You have not felt depressed or down, just somewhat lonely.

Ideas, concerns and expectations – You think the dizziness may just be your 'nerves' as you have not been yourself since your good friend Edna died 6 months ago. You miss her and feel more anxious about your own health, and have started to think more and more about your own mortality. You are also concerned that you might fall and that you are on your own. You want the doctor to sort you out and solve all these problems for you. But if you feel confident in the doctor and he or she explains that it is unlikely to be anything serious and probably, as you suspect, down to your nerves, you will be able to accept this. You feel that you take enough tablets as it is, and do not want to take any more. But you are happy to have some blood tests and see the doctor again.

First words spoken to doctor – 'I've been getting ever so dizzy, doctor, over the last few months, I wonder if it's to do with my nerves. I want you to sort me out.'

Medical history – You had a heart attack 10 years ago from which you made a good recovery. You also suffer from osteoarthritis in your hips and knees.

Drug history – You take various tablets following your heart attack, including aspirin 75 mg once a day ('to help thin the blood'), bisoprolol 5 mg once a day ('to help the heart'), ramipril 2.5 mg once a day (you are not sure why you take this) and simvastatin

40 mg at night ('to help the cholesterol'). You take an occasional paracetamol for pains in your hips and knees.

Social history – You have lived on your own since your husband died 15 years ago and have never required any home help, other than your daughter who visits several times a week and takes you shopping. Since your friend died you go out much less frequently. You used to do everything together – bingo, dancing, lunch clubs and bowls – but it just does not seem the same going on your own, and you worry about falling with the dizzy spells. You smoked 20 cigarettes a day for over 30 years, but stopped about 10 years before your heart attack. You have the odd glass of sherry on special occasions. You do not drive.

Family history – There are no major medical problems in your immediate family.

- Having read the information given to the simulated patient, what do you now think this station is testing?
- Make notes or discuss your thoughts with a colleague before you turn the page.

Review your approach to this station:

Tested at this station:

1. Encouraging patients to take responsibility for their health and well-being.
2. History-taking skills.
3. Physical examination.
4. Managing uncertainty.

Domain 1 – Interpersonal skills

Encouraging patients to take responsibility for their health and well-being (overlap with domain 3)

Patients often present to their surgery expecting the doctor to 'fix' whatever problems they have, whether they are medically related or not. Encouraging patients to take some responsibility and to adopt self-help measures, where appropriate and with support, is a key skill that you should be able to demonstrate:

- This patient has a number of problems – loneliness, grief, anxiety, worries about falling and being on her own, and dizziness. She will try to place the responsibility for dealing with these problems on you, and expects you to provide solutions.
- Although you may be able to help, it is important to explain to the patient that there is much that she can do to address these issues herself (see Managing uncertainty below).
- One response to the patient's opening statement might be: *'Well, let's discuss this further and see what we can both do to try to improve things.'* This signals that she, too, will need to take on some responsibility.
- In this case you may feel under particular pressure to 'solve' the patient's various problems, as her daughter is one of your colleagues at the practice. But by encouraging the patient to tackle some of these issues herself, you can empower her to be an active agent in her own health promotion.

Domain 2 – Data gathering, technical and assessment skills

History-taking skills

You need to take a focused history to try to identify the cause of her dizziness. But remember that you will score more marks and obtain key details if you start with open questions and elicit the patient's ideas, concerns and expectations before moving on to more specific, closed questions:

- She is getting dizzy and thinks this may be due to her 'nerves'. Can she say more about this?
- What are her thoughts about what is going on?
- Does she have any particular concerns about these symptoms?
- What was she hoping would happen from coming to see the doctor today?
- 'Dizziness' is an imprecise term that needs to be clarified. Does she mean that she feels faint at certain times or is she describing a sensation of movement, e.g. spinning, when there is none?
- What is she doing when she gets these dizzy spells? Has she just stood up or moved her head?

- Any problems with her ears? Any ringing or deafness?
- Does she vomit or feel nauseous when she feels dizzy?
- Any palpitations or chest pain?
- Any similar symptoms to when she had her heart attack?
- Does she smoke?
- She mentions her 'nerves'. What has her mood been like recently? Has she felt low? Do any situations make her feel anxious?
- Does she find herself breathing faster when the dizziness comes on? Does she feel anxious first and then dizzy?
- Has she fallen or banged her head recently?
- Has she blacked out or lost consciousness?
- Any weakness or numbness in her arms or legs? Any visual problems?
- Is her neck stiff or sore?
- Has she had a cough recently or pain passing urine? Has she been feverish?
- Does she drive?

Physical examination

Although there is a lot to cover at this station, do not neglect to examine the patient. You will be expected to examine her ears and perform a brief cardiovascular examination (see below). You will subsequently be told that there are no abnormal findings. If you indicate that you wish to perform further examinations, such as a full neurological examination, neck movements or Hallpike test (positional manoeuvre to induce vertigo), you will be informed that this is not necessary and to assume that the findings are normal.

- The patient is complaining of dizziness and has a history of cardiovascular disease.
- As part of a brief cardiovascular examination you would be expected to examine her:
  - pulse
  - Blood pressure (BP), including checking for a postural drop
  - carotids for any bruits
  - heart sounds at the four standard precordium sites: mitral, tricuspid, pulmonary and aortic areas.
- You may be tempted to perform a more thorough cardiovascular examination (see Further reading below), however there is limited time for the consultation and what is expected is a focused examination.

Domain 3 – Clinical management skills

Managing uncertainty

One of the specific problem-solving competencies, as set out in the GP curriculum, is the ability to manage conditions that may present in an undifferentiated way. You are expected to be able to demonstrate when you can reassure patients, when expectant management is appropriate ('watchful waiting') and when you need to initiate diagnostic tests or treatment – taking into account the patient's wishes. In this case, the cause of the patient's dizziness is not completely clear from the history and examination findings today:

- This is a deliberately complex and challenging station. The patient presents with several issues: the feelings of loss for her friend, increasing anxiety over her own health, and episodes of lightheadedness with no clear diagnostic pattern. Additionally, she wants you to take responsibility for her problems and to solve them for her.
- In a 10-minute consultation you need to be able to elicit her agenda, take a focused history and examination to try to help diagnose the cause of her dizziness, and offer her management options that are acceptable to both you and the patient. You also need to try to get her to take on some responsibility for her problems.
- This is unlikely to be a one-off consultation with the patient and you need to think about what would be most appropriate – and safe – to do at this first meeting.
- You might be tempted to send her for a range of investigations, including blood tests, 24-hour BP monitoring, 24-hour electrocardiogram (ECG) recording, tilt test, magnetic resonance imaging (MRI) scan of her head and neck x-rays, or even to refer her to an elderly care specialist today. However, if you suspect that her symptoms are related to anxiety and grief, then providing support and advice should be your main priority, together with incremental investigations, as a more appropriate way forward.
- You can reassure the patient that there are no worrying findings on examination. Explain that you are unsure of the exact diagnosis, although, as she suggests, the dizziness may be related to her anxieties and grief at the loss of her friend.
- Given the uncertainty about the diagnosis, her age and medical history, you would be expected to organize some preliminary blood tests – e.g. full blood count (FBC), urea and electrolytes (U&Es), glucose and thyroid function tests (TFTs) – and arrange to review the results with her. Is she happy with this plan?
- Various self-help management options which you could suggest include:
  - having her eyes tested at the optician
  - attending a local bereavement group or bereavement counselling
  - considering a pendant alarm to wear to allay her anxieties about falling at home
  - thinking about whether she would feel safer and enjoy the company provided by sheltered accommodation
  - perhaps trying to go along to the groups she used to attend, or accessing befriending/buddy support services through organizations such as Age Concern or Help the Aged
  - perhaps asking her daughter to take her out more.
- You could also offer a trial of a vestibular sedative such as cinnarizine 30 mg TDS or prochlorperazine 5 mg TDS. However, the *British National Formulary* makes clear that when considering prescribing for the elderly, non-pharmacological approaches are often preferred to treat lightheadedness, sleeplessness and headache when these are related to life events or social stressors, e.g. in widowhood and loneliness. Moreover, the patient is not keen to take any more medication and you should respect this.
- Safety netting – make sure the patient knows what to do if she develops any new symptoms, such as chest pain or blackouts.

- The key to managing uncertainty is to ensure that whatever plan is agreed, it is acceptable to both doctor and patient. Is she happy with the advice about sources of help, that you are doing some basic tests, and that you will review things in 2 weeks, or sooner if required?

Knowledge base

References: RCGP curriculum statement 15.7, NHS Clinical Knowledge Summaries, Colledge *et al.*, *BMJ* – see Further reading below.

	Causes of dizziness

Otological	• Peripheral
	   • vestibular neuritis
	   • Ménière's disease (vertigo, tinnitus, deafness)
	   • benign paroxysmal positional vertigo (BPPV)
	   • Ramsay Hunt syndrome
	• Central
	• Acoustic neuroma

Psychological	• Anxiety • Hyperventilation
Cardiovascular	• Arrhythmias • Postural hypotension

Neurological	• Stroke
	   • brainstem or cerebellar
	   • haemorrhage or infarction
	• Trauma and concussion
	• Peripheral neuropathy
	• Multiple sclerosis
	• Parkinsonism
	• Brain tumours
	• Multisystem atrophy
	• Migraneous vertigo

Drugs	• Anti-hypertensives • Vasodilators • Anti-depressants • Parkinson's disease medication (e.g. levodopa, selegiline) • Phosphodiesterase-5 inhibitors (e.g. sildenafil)
Other	• Poor vision • Cervical spondylosis • Hypoglycaemia

Take-home messages

- In general practice, conditions often present in an undifferentiated way. You need to be comfortable dealing with diagnostic uncertainty.
- Encourage patients to take responsibility for their health and well-being, with appropriate support and advice.
- Physical examinations needs to be slick and focused given the limited time in the Clinical Skills Assessment Clinical Skills Assessment (CSA).

Algorithm for evaluation of the cause of dizziness in elderly patients in general practice. From Colledge NR *et al.* Evaluation of investigations to diagnose the cause of dizziness in elderly people: a community based controlled study. *BMJ* 1996; 313: 788–792. Reproduced with permission from BMJ Publishing Group.

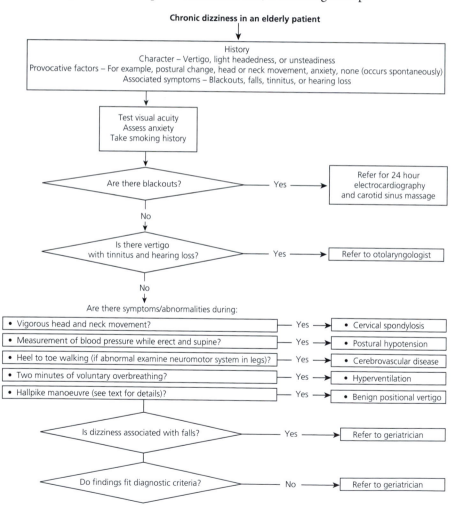

Tasks

- Re-run the scenario with the patient describing 'blackouts' when she feels dizzy. How might this change what management options you would offer?
- Re-run the scenario with you finding (or being told by the CSA examiner) that the patient has an irregularly irregular pulse. How would you explain this to the patient and how might this change what management options you would offer?
- Re-run the scenario with the patient having recently returned from a trip to South Africa.

1-minute explanations for patients

- Explain to a patient what BPPV is.
- Explain to a patient how emotions and feelings can sometimes manifest themselves as physical symptoms.
- Explain to a patient why you would usually listen to her neck for carotid bruits.

Ideas for further revision

The simulated patients in the CSA will be similar to those you encounter in an ordinary GP surgery and so you would be wise to take common presenting conditions – such as dizziness, back pain, headaches, indigestion, irregular periods, pill requests, abdominal pain, etc. – and ensure that for each of these you have a mental checklist for history taking, examination and management options. In the international setting (e.g. those candidates undertaking MRCGP[INT]) such a common presentation as dizziness is equally relevant. Role-play the scenario, changing the patient details to suit your local context.

Further reading

Colledge NR, Barr-Hamilton RM, Lewis SJ, Sellar RJ, Wilson JA. Evaluation of investigations to diagnose the cause of dizziness in elderly people: a community based controlled study. *BMJ* 1996; 313: 788–792 www.bmj.com

Kanagalingam J, Hajioff D, Bennett S. 10-minute consultation: vertigo. *BMJ* 2005; 330: 523 www.bmj.com

NHS Clinical Knowledge Summaries: vertigo www.cks.nhs.uk/vertigo

RCGP curriculum statement 15.7 – Clinical management: neurological problems www.rcgp-curriculum.org.uk/PDF/curr_15_7_Neurological_problems.pdf

Thomas J, Monaghan T. *Oxford Handbook of Clinical Examination and Practical Skills*. Oxford: Oxford University Press, 2007

STATION 10

Information given to candidates

Zoë Brighthouse is a 16-year-old patient whose parents and older sister are also registered with the practice.

Her records show that she attended the surgery a week ago with her mother and saw one of the Foundation Year 2 doctors.

At that time she was complaining of a week's history of sore throat and general malaise. Examination is documented as:

Chest	Clear
Otoscopy	Normal
Throat	?Exudate on tonsils
Neck	Enlarged lymph nodes anterior cervical chain

She was prescribed 1 week's course of amoxicillin 500 mg TDS for ?tonsillitis

She had been prescribed amoxicillin for an ear infection earlier in the year without any problems.

The patient is on her own today.

As the patient enters the room she says, 'I've stopped those tablets the other doctor gave me because they made me come out in a rash.'

- What do you think this station is testing?
- Make notes or discuss your thoughts with a colleague before you read on.

Plan your approach to this station:

Information given to simulated patient

Basic details – You are Zoë Brighthouse, a Caucasian 16-year-old pupil at the local state school.

Appearance and behaviour – You are quiet and take a while to open up to the doctor. But if you feel that the doctor has a caring and understanding manner, then you are more likely to be forthcoming earlier on in the consultation about your true concerns about HIV (see Ideas, concerns and expectations).

History

Freely divulged to doctor – You have been feeling 'awful' for a couple of weeks now with a sore throat, fever, general aches and pains and tiredness. Last week you saw one of the other doctors at the practice with your mother and you were prescribed antibiotics for a throat infection. The same day you started the tablets you came out in a fine red rash all over your body, so you have not taken any more. The rash has now settled. You were not able to book an earlier appointment than today.

Divulged to doctor if specifically asked – You have only missed 3 days of school in the last 2 weeks. You have not had a cough or brought up any phlegm. You have not vomited and you have not suffered from diarrhoea or constipation. You have not had any abdominal pain or pain passing urine. You are not going to the toilet to urinate more frequently and you do not have excessive thirst. Two weeks ago you had vaginal sex with a boy from your class who you do not know very well, after a party at the home of a friend. You did not have oral sex. It was the first time you had ever had sex. You asked him to use a condom – which he did – as you are not on the pill and were worried about getting pregnant. You do not think there were any problems such as the condom splitting. You only had a couple of drinks that night and felt in control of the situation. The sex was consensual. You have not had any genital symptoms, such as itchiness or a discharge. You have never had any genital infections. You did a pregnancy test last week, 'just to make sure', which was negative. Your periods are always regular and you started your period on time 4 days ago. You did not tell the doctor last week about having had sex as your mother was with you.

Ideas, concerns and expectations – You are upset with yourself as you had planned not to have sex until you were older, with someone you loved. You think that the tablets probably did cause the rash but read on the internet that when you are infected with HIV you can develop an illness with general aches and pains, a sore throat and a rash – just like your symptoms. Even though you used a condom when you had sex, you are still worried that you could have got a sexually transmitted infection, such as HIV. You have heard of condoms splitting without people knowing and this has been preying on your mind. You have never wanted to take the oral contraception pill or any hormonal alternatives as you 'don't want to put all those hormones in your body'. You want advice from the doctor on the chances of you having HIV and whether you should have an HIV test.

First words spoken to doctor – 'I've stopped those tablets the other doctor gave me because they made me come out in a rash.'

Medical history – You had eczema as a child but are no longer affected by this. You rarely go to see the doctor as you are generally fit and well. You had an ear infection earlier this year which settled with antibiotics.

Drug history – You do not take any regular medication and took only one of the antibiotic tablets the doctor prescribed last week. You took the same antibiotic (amoxicillin) for an ear infection earlier this year without any problems. As far as you know you are not allergic to any medication. You do not use any illicit drugs.

Social history – You live with your parents and sister who is 1 year older than you. You are doing well at school and have GCSE exams coming up at the end of this academic year. You are popular at school and have a close group of friends. You have the odd cigarette when you are out but you do not really like smoking. You are sensible about drinking alcohol – you never get really drunk – but you do drink several alcopops when you go out with your friends at the weekend.

Family history – There are no major health problems in your family.

- Having read the information given to the simulated patient, what do you now think this station is testing?
- Make notes or discuss your thoughts with a colleague before you turn the page.

Review your approach to this station:

Tested at this station:

1. Identifying a hidden agenda.
2. History taking from a reticent patient.
3. Physical examination.
4. Reaching a shared management plan with an adolescent.

Domain 1 – Interpersonal skills

Identifying a hidden agenda

Patients often present with a problem that is not the main reason for their attendance at the surgery. You need to be open to the possibility of such hidden agendas and allow the patient every opportunity to disclose his or her true concerns:

- It can be daunting for a teenager to see a doctor on their own. To create the right environment for her to open up you need to employ excellent communication skills through active listening, showing empathy and encouraging her to contribute as an equal partner in the consultation.
- Your attitude to anything she tells you about her health or health concerns must be non-judgemental and supportive. Patients often test you out early on in the consultation to see if you are the sort of doctor they feel happy to disclose more personal information to.
- Pick up on any clues that the patient may give, e.g. *'You seem very anxious about what has happened. Do you think there might be something else going on other than a throat infection?'*
- Stay patient-focused and if you feel there is a mismatch between your worries about the presenting complaint and the patient's, then explore her ideas, concerns and expectations further.

Domain 2 – Data gathering, technical and assessment skills

History taking from a reticent patient

There is the potential for this scenario to be challenging in terms of time management, as the patient is initially slow in giving a history. But if she feels that you have a caring and understanding manner, she is more likely to offer the information you need to safely manage the consultation while also addressing her agenda:

- You could ask whether the patient came with anyone today, e.g. she may have a friend in the waiting room. If so, would she like them to come in to give her some support?
- If during the consultation you suspect that she may want to disclose further information but seems reluctant, remind her that your discussion is confidential.
- Ask her to recap on what has happened over the last couple of weeks, as this allows you to find out her understanding of events, including last week's visit to see your colleague.
- Ask about any allergies to medication. Check that when she was prescribed amoxicillin for an ear infection earlier in the year she did not have any similar reaction.

- The clear history from the notes, together with the information about a rash starting soon after taking the antibiotics, should alert you early on to the probable diagnosis of infectious mononucleosis (glandular fever).
- However, be careful not to close down the consultation early, and ensure that you still ask questions about her health beliefs, concerns and expectations, or you will miss the key element to this scenario – namely, the patient's anxiety about possible HIV infection.
- Allow the patient time to discuss her concerns regarding having had sex and her worries about HIV infection.
- You should take a full sexual history (see Station 5) to assess HIV risk.
- Use words that the patient can understand – do not assume that what you might consider simple terms, e.g. 'vagina', are readily understood.
- Given her age it is also important to find out whether the sex was consensual. Enquire about the age of her sexual partner. If he was significantly older then you might be worried that there was an element of coercion.
- Has she been able to discuss her worries with anyone else, either friends or family?

Physical examination

If you say you would like to examine the patient, you will be told that this is not necessary and to assume that the findings are the same as when she was seen last week (see Information given to candidates).

Domain 3 – Clinical management skills

Reaching a shared management plan with an adolescent (overlap with domain 1)

In addition to reassuring the patient over her main concern – the risk of HIV infection – this consultation is an opportunity to cover wider health promotion issues:

- You should explain how the history suggests a diagnosis of glandular fever, although she would need a blood test to confirm this. You can reassure her that this is a common condition, caused by a virus (Epstein-Barr) and is usually a short, self-limiting illness, although it can run a protracted course in some cases. You can explain how it is spread – by saliva – and therefore she should avoid kissing and sharing cups and towels while she is still unwell.
- Advise rest, plenty of fluids and simple painkillers, such as paracetamol and ibuprofen, together with self-help measures such as gargling with salt water for her sore throat.
- Is she happy to have some blood taken to confirm the diagnosis (full blood count (FBC) to look for leucocytosis and monospot)?
- Reassure her that as she has just had her period and the pregnancy test was negative, she can feel confident that she is not pregnant.
- Reassure her that her risk of HIV would be assessed as low, as she had protected sex, and there would therefore be little indication for having an HIV test. What does she think about this?

- If, despite your reassurances, she feels that for peace of mind she would still like to have an HIV test, you should advise her that she should have a repeat test in 3 months as even with the standard combined antigen and antibody HIV test, it can still take up to 3 months to become positive. In the interim she should use condoms.
- Be positive about her proven ability to negotiate practising safer sex – using a condom – and encourage continued use. Advise her where she can get these herself rather than having to rely on a partner. Often there are local resources such as a Young People's Project, Teenage Health Bus, or schemes such as C-card where teenagers can show a card at genitourinary medicine (GUM) or family planning clinics to get free condoms, without the embarrassment of having to ask a receptionist or pharmacist.
- Has she considered other forms of contraception, such as long-acting reversible contraceptives, e.g. the Nexplanon® implant?
- Offer information on sexual health screening services at GUM clinics or at the surgery, e.g. swabs or a urine sample to screen for infections such as chlamydia. Does she know anything about these sorts of services?
- The GP curriculum states that every consultation with a child or young person should be an opportunity for general health promotion advice. How much exercise does she do? What is her diet like? Does she use alcohol or illicit drugs? Are there any small steps she could realistically take to make her lifestyle healthier?
- Encourage her to discuss what has happened with her parents or sister. If she does not feel comfortable speaking to her family, is there any other adult she could talk to, such as a teacher, school nurse or youth worker she trusts?
- Remember to negotiate all the above with the patient rather than simply telling her what steps she can take.
- Check her understanding at regular intervals during the consultation and ask her to explain the plan you have jointly agreed back to you.

Knowledge base – Children, consent, confidentiality and the law

References: GMC 2007, House of Lords *Gillick* case, and Family Law Reform Act 1969 – see Further reading below.

	English law
Under 16 years old	• The House of Lord's judgment in the *Gillick* case (see Further reading below) ruled that the consent of a child under 16 can, in certain circumstances, have legal effect. This applies even if the parents disagree with the child over the proposed treatment. • Lord Scarman held that a test of capacity be applied, which could determine whether the young person had 'sufficient understanding and intelligence to enable him or her to understand fully what is proposed' (*Gillick* judgment p. 423). • This has become known as *Gillick*-competence. • However, patients under 16 who are *Gillick*-competent should still be encouraged to involve their parents.

(continued)

continued

	English law
16 and 17 years old	• Although all those aged under 18 are classed as minors, the Family Law Reform Act 1969 gives statutory recognition to the consent of 16 and 17 year olds to any 'surgical, medical or dental treatment', making it 'as effective as it would be if he were of full age' (sections 8(1) and 8(3)). • In other words, those aged 16 and 17 are presumed to have the competence to give consent for themselves.
≥18 years old	• Treated as adults under the law, i.e. presumed to be competent.
Emergencies	• As with adults, if a patient under 18 is not competent, e.g. if they are unconscious, and it is an emergency situation such that it is unreasonable to wait, then you are legally entitled to treat without consent, acting in the best interests of the patient.
Consent versus refusal	• As the law currently stands, minors – namely, all those under 18 years of age – are legally entitled to *consent* to medical treatment (so long as they are *Gillick*-competent if under 16), yet they do not have an absolute right to *refuse* medical treatment. This is because anyone with parental responsibility can legally give consent on behalf of a minor. • However, in practice, it would be highly unlikely for a doctor to proceed with an intervention in the face of a competent child's refusal, even if the consent of someone with parental responsibility did technically mean that there was legal consent. This situation would require further discussion and potential involvement of the courts.
Confidentiality	• You must keep confidential any information a competent child asks you not to disclose, unless you believe doing so would put the child or others at risk of serious harm. • You should encourage the patient to involve their family, unless this is not in their best interests. • You should consult with a senior colleague and your defence organization before taking the significant step of breaking confidentiality.

Fraser guidelines	• In the *Gillick* judgment, Lord Fraser listed criteria that must be met to allow doctors to lawfully give contraceptive advice and treatment to children under 16 without parental involvement:
	  • the young person understands the advice
	  • the young person cannot be persuaded to involve their parents
	  • the young person is likely to begin or continue having sex with or without contraceptive treatment
	  • the young person's physical or mental health, or both, is likely to suffer unless they receive treatment
	  • the young person's best interests require them to have contraceptive advice or treatment without parental consent.

Take-home messages
- The key skill when dealing with adolescents and young people is treating them as real partners in the consultation.
- Picking up on cues from the patient will help identify hidden agendas.
- Signposting patients to support services and other agencies is important within primary care.

Tasks

- Re-run the scenario with the patient aged 15 years. How might this change your approach?
- Re-run the scenario with the patient aged 15 years and the male she has had sex with being 38 years old. What would now be the main focus of this scenario?
- Run a scenario where Zoë's mother has come to see you a week later. Her mother says, 'I know Zoë came to see you last week and I want to know what's going on.' How would you approach this consultation?

1-minute explanations for patients

- Explain how the contraceptive implant works.
- Explain what a sexual health 'check-up' might involve.
- Explain the limits of confidentiality (e.g. see the second task above).

Ideas for further revision

Although this station was not specifically about consent issues in children, you could easily be presented in the Clinical Skills assessment (CSA) with either a child or parent of a child under 16 years of age who has requested contraception or an abortion. Make sure you feel happy about how you would deal with such a situation and that you are familiar with the law and national guidance in this area.

Further reading

0–18 years: guidance for all doctors. GMC, London 2007 www.gmc-uk.org/guidance/ethical_guidance/children_guidance_index.asp

Gillick v West Norfolk and Wisbech Area Health Authority and another [1985] 3 All ER 402

NHS Clinical Knowledge Summaries: HIV www.cks.nhs.uk/hiv_infection_and_aids

NHS Clinical Knowledge Summaries: glandular fever www.cks.nhs.uk/glandular_fever

NICE – Prevention of sexually transmitted infections and under 18 conceptions. Public health intervention guidance 3. Quick reference guide, February 2007 http://guidance.nice.org.uk/PH3/QuickRefGuide/pdf/English

RCGP curriculum statement 8 – Care of children and young people www.rcgp-curriculum.org.uk/PDF/curr_8_Care_of_Children_and_Young_People.pdf

The Terrence Higgins Trust – the leading HIV and AIDS charity in the UK www.tht.org.uk

'You're Welcome': quality criteria for young people friendly health services. London: Department of Health, 2011 www.dh.gov.uk/en/Publicationsandstatistics/Publications/PublicationsPolicyAndGuidance/DH_126813

Information given to candidates

Michelle McKinley is a 20-year-old shop assistant who recently registered with your surgery. She saw the practice nurse for a new patient check and her records state:

- Smoker – 10 cigarettes a day
- Alcohol – approximately 8 units a week
- Exercise – minimal
- Urinalysis – normal
- Blood pressure – 122/76 mmHg
- Height 1.52 m; weight 72 kg; body mass index (BMI) = 31 kg/m^2
- Just moved to the area with husband
- No children
- Taking folic acid 400 µg OD as trying to get pregnant

The first words the patient says as she enters the room are, 'I've been trying to get pregnant for 6 months now but nothing seems to be happening, doctor.'

- What do you think this station is testing?
- Make notes opposite or discuss your thoughts with a colleague before you turn the page.

Plan your approach to this station:

Information given to simulated patient

Basic details – You are Michelle McKinley, a Caucasian 20-year-old shop assistant.

Appearance and behaviour – You are casually dressed and come across as a little anxious. You speak very matter-of-factly about sex and your efforts to get pregnant.

History

Freely divulged to doctor – You were married 6 months ago and have been trying to become pregnant since then. You were living with your parents-in-law until last month when you and your husband moved into a rented flat in the neighbouring town. You do not understand why you are not pregnant yet as your friends seem to be able to fall pregnant as soon as they stop taking the pill. You thought you should see the doctor to find out whether you needed some tests.

Divulged to doctor if specifically asked – It was difficult when you were living in a room at your parents-in-law to have the privacy to have sexual intercourse regularly, but you still managed to do so at least once a week. For the last couple of months you have been trying to have lots of sex in the 5-day period right in the middle between your periods, as your mum said this was the best time to get pregnant. But doing this is making both you and your husband rather stressed and feeling 'under pressure', such that sex has now become more of a chore. Your periods were always regular – every 28 days – before you started on the pill (back when you were 16 years old) and have returned to this pattern within a couple of months of stopping the pill 6 months ago. You have never had heavy periods or bleeding in between periods. You do not have any vaginal discharge. You have never had any sexually transmitted infections (STIs) and before you met your husband had only two previous boyfriends with whom you had sex. You are having penetrative vaginal sex (your husband is putting his penis into your vagina and ejaculating sperm). You do not have excessive facial hair. Your weight is steady.

Ideas, concerns and expectations – You thought that as soon as you stopped taking the pill you would get pregnant. You know that sometimes older women take a while to get pregnant, but at your age you do not understand why there seems to be a 'problem'. Your mum said it could be your 'hormones' and you should see the doctor. You think the 'problem' must be your fault, as your husband was able to get a previous girlfriend pregnant, although she had an abortion. You have a sketchy idea of what happens each month when your body produces an egg and how that fits in with you having a period, but you would feel 'stupid' if you asked. If the doctor comes across as kind and understanding and reassures you that there is nothing to worry about, you will be happy with the consultation. You will try to take on board any general health advice the doctor gives you to help increase the chance of you becoming pregnant.

First words spoken to doctor – 'I've been trying to get pregnant for 6 months now but nothing seems to be happening, doctor.'

Medical history – You know that you are a little overweight and should give up smoking, but otherwise you think of yourself as fairly healthy. You have never had any medical problems, apart from the odd ear or throat infection. You have never had an abortion or miscarriage, or ever been pregnant.

Drug history – You have been taking 400 µg of folic acid once a day for 6 months. Before you were married you used Microgynon 30 – 'the combined pill' – for contraception, which you started when you were 16 years old. You are not allergic to any medication.

Social history – For the last month you have been living with your husband, who has just qualified as an electrician, in rented accommodation. Prior to that you lived with your parents-in-law. You and your husband both smoke about 10 cigarettes a day. You drink about four cans of normal-strength lager over a week. You left school when you were 16 years old with four GCSE qualifications. You work as an assistant in a high street clothes shop.

Family history – There is no history of major health problems or infertility in your family. As far as you know, no one has polycystic ovaries or had an early menopause.

- Having read the information given to the simulated patient, what do you now think this station is testing?
- Make notes or discuss your thoughts with a colleague before you turn the page.

Review your approach to this station:

Tested at this station:

1. History-taking skills.
2. Offering reassurance.
3. Health promotion around fertility issues.

Domain 1 – Data gathering, technical and assessment skills

History-taking skills

Simply from the patient's opening words you may feel that there is nothing to worry about here. But it is important to understand the patient's perspective on events and why she has attended now. You also need to exclude symptoms that would prompt investigation even at this early stage. Questions you could ask include:

- Why is she concerned about not being pregnant yet?
- What are her expectations on how long it takes to get pregnant?
- What is her experience of family and friends trying to conceive?
- What does her husband think about this?
- Did she and her husband use any form of contraception before they started trying for a baby?
- How long after stopping the combined pill did it take for her periods to return?
- Any previous pregnancies, miscarriages, terminations or pelvic surgery?
- Any previous STIs?
- Has she had any abdominal pains? Or vaginal discharge?
- Are her periods regular? Any bleeding between periods? Is her bleeding heavy?
- How often are they having sex? Is it vaginal sex?
- Is she still smoking? How much alcohol is she currently drinking?
- Does she take any regular medication, or over-the-counter or illicit drugs?
- Any family history of similar problems or early menopause?
- Does her husband have any children from previous relationships? Or has he ever made someone pregnant?
- What type of work does she do? And her husband? Some occupational agents can have an effect on both women's and men's fertility – see National Institute for Health and Clinical Excellence (NICE) guideline reference.
- Does she know whether she had a rubella vaccination when she was younger?

Domain 2 – Interpersonal skills

Offering reassurance

This patient has been trying to get pregnant for only 6 months and there is nothing in the history suggesting an underlying problem. The key here is to recognize her presentation as normal, explain this to the patient and try to reassure her, and then to go on to offer health promotion advice about trying to conceive:

- The patient has an unrealistic expectation of how long it normally takes to conceive. You could make clear that it is not unusual, even for normal healthy couples, to take over a year, or longer, to conceive (see Knowledge base).

- The patient and her husband have been trying for only 6 months and for the majority of that time it was difficult to have regular sex due to living with her parents-in-law.
- Also, it can take a few months after stopping the pill before the body returns to a normal hormonal cycle.
- However, she is now having regular periods, which suggests that she is ovulating – *'producing an egg that can join up with a sperm to make an embryo which grows into a baby'*. A diagram might help her understanding.
- As she and her husband have found out, it can be stressful trying to have sex at particular times each month. You should advise her that this is not necessary and they should just try to have regular sexual intercourse – about two to three times a week.
- You should explain that they (and it should ideally be both of them) need to come back to the surgery only if she is still not pregnant after a year in total of trying.

Domain 3 – Clinical management skills

Health promotion around fertility issues

You should use this opportunity to discuss lifestyle issues such as smoking, alcohol, diet, exercise and weight loss, which could all help increase the patient's chance of becoming pregnant, while also promoting general good health:

- Stopping smoking would be of huge benefit to her health, may increase her chance of conceiving and is important for a healthy pregnancy. Might this be something she and her husband would consider doing together so that the home environment becomes a smoke-free zone for their future child?
- Advise her that the latest recommendations advise that women significantly limit their alcohol intake when trying to conceive. Does she think she would be able to do this?
- Women with a BMI of more than 29 kg/m^2 are likely to take longer to conceive. You could discuss this with the patient and look at ways she might address this, including through her diet and taking more exercise.
- You have given the patient a lot of information today. If she has any further questions, or wants to talk more about this, perhaps next time she could bring her husband, too.

Knowledge base – Infertility

(*References*: National Institute for Health and Clinical Excellence (NICE) guideline. Fertility: assessment and treatment for people with fertility problems (update). Draft guidance for consultation. May 2012 (definitive update of earlier 2004 guidance due Oct 2012). www.nice.org.uk)

Infertility:

Defined pragmatically as the period of time people have been trying to conceive without success after which formal investigation is justified and possible treatment implemented.

Early referral for specialist consultation if:

- Known cause of infertility or history of predisposing factors for infertility
- Woman's age ≥36 years
- People with HIV, hepatitis B and hepatitis C
- Prior treatment for cancer.

Initial advice for people concerned about delays in conception:

- Inform people that more than 80% of couples in the general population will conceive within 1 year if:
  - the woman is aged less than 40 years, and
  - they do not use contraception and have regular sexual intercourse.
- Lifestyle advice:
  - vaginal sexual intercourse every 2–3 days
  - ≤1–2 units alcohol once or twice a week for women reduces the risk of harming the foetus; ≤3–4 units/day for men is unlikely to affect semen quality
  - smoking cessation programme for smokers
  - body mass index of 19–29 kg/m^2
  - information about prescribed, over-the-counter and recreational drugs
  - information about occupational hazards
- Offer preconceptional advice:
  - folic acid
  - rubella susceptibility and cervical screening.

Principles of care:

- Couple-centred management.
- Access to evidence-based information (verbal and written or audiovisual Material).
- Counselling from someone not directly involved in management of the individual's and/or the couple's fertility problems.
- Contact with fertility support groups.
- Specialist team input.

Take-home messages

- Patients' understanding of what constitutes 'normal' can be unrealistic.
- Patient education and providing reassurance are key roles for the GP.
- Use every opportunity for health promotion.

Tasks

- Re-run the scenario with the patient returning having been trying to conceive for 18 months. How would this change your management? What investigations would you consider?
- Re-run the scenario with an Asian couple attending, with the husband anxious that 'something must be done' regarding the fact that his wife is not pregnant 6 months after their arranged marriage.

- Re-run the scenario with the patient returning wanting a termination of a pregnancy, as she split up from her husband and has become pregnant following a casual sexual encounter.

1-minute explanations for patients

- Explain the normal menstrual cycle, including when ovulation occurs.
- Explain the procedure for providing a semen sample.

Ideas for further revision

It is easy to dismiss those who present when there is no medical abnormality as the 'worried well'. However, as healthcare professionals we should see patient education and providing reassurance as key parts of our role. These consultations also offer an opportunity to give healthy lifestyle advice. In your day-to-day surgeries, try to regularly offer such advice, such that this becomes almost second nature. Simple health-promotion strategies, such as encouraging smoking cessation, can offer patients extremely cost-effective interventions. This scenario can be adapted to acknowledge different cultural expectations.

Further reading

Infertility Network UK. Advice and support for those dealing with fertility problems www.infertilitynetworkuk.com

NHS Clinical Knowledge Summaries: infertility www.cks.nhs.uk/infertility

NICE guideline. Fertility: assessment and treatment for people with fertility problems (update). Draft guidance for consultation. May 2012 (definitive update of earlier 2004 guidance due October 2012) www.nice.org.uk

RCGP curriculum statement 10.1 – Women's health www.rcgp-curriculum.org.uk/PDF/curr_10_1_Womens_Health.pdf

Information given to candidates

Candidates note: this station is a **telephone consultation** with a patient. Please answer the telephone when it rings. The examiner will not enter your room, but will be able to hear both you and the patient.

Miranda Rogerson is a 42-year-old female patient with Crohn's disease.

She has been under the care of the gastroenterologists for 4 years.

The last clinic letter from 1 month ago states:

Dear GP,

Mrs Rogerson is currently stable on azathioprine 125 mg OD. However, she has had three admissions in the last year with flare-ups of her colonic inflammatory Crohn's disease and her last colonoscopy revealed a well-defined region in the proximal ascending colon. We have discussed with Mrs Rogerson that surgery will probably be the next option, if things flare up again, although we would of course reassess at that time.

The patient's GP surgery, where you are based, is in London.

The first thing the patient says when you pick up the phone is, 'Hello doctor, it's Miranda Rogerson here. I'm away on business at the moment in Aberdeen and the Crohn's seems to be flaring up.'

- What do you think this station is testing?
- Make notes or discuss your thoughts with a colleague before you read on.

Plan your approach to this station:

Information given to simulated patient

Basic details – You are Miranda Rogerson, a Caucasian 42-year-old management consultant currently on a week-long visit to one of your clients in Aberdeen. You are ringing your GP surgery back in London for advice. You suffer from Crohn's disease (an inflammatory condition affecting your bowels) which seems to have flared up in the last 3 days.

Appearance and behaviour – You come across on the telephone as articulate and intelligent. Initially you underplay the severity of your symptoms to try to persuade the doctor – and yourself – that you can wait until you return home before you see someone.

History

Freely divulged to doctor – You have Crohn's disease and see the specialist team at your local hospital in London every 4 months. Things have been fairly settled since you were last discharged from hospital 4 months ago, after a week's stay. You take regular medication to 'keep on top of the Crohn's'. You have not been feeling too good for 3 days, with diarrhoea and tummy pains.

Divulged to doctor if specifically asked – Yesterday you opened your bowels six times, and today you have been eight times already. The rectal bleeding you get when your Crohn's flares up is back and now pretty heavy (you have used four pads so far today). Your appetite has been poor for a couple of weeks and you have lost about 4 kg over that time. You have felt generally 'washed out' over the last week. You were feeling hot last night and have taken plenty of paracetamol, but still feel feverish today. The abdominal pains are on the right-hand side, lower down, and it is particularly tender in that area. One of your colleagues said you were looking rather pale yesterday. You have not had any joint or eye problems.

Ideas, concerns and expectations – The work in Aberdeen is a key contract and you see it as a real opportunity to show your boss that you are ready for promotion. You feel that if you have to leave before the end of the week it will not look good to your seniors. You know that your Crohn's is worse, but you are hoping that you can hold out until the end of the trip. However, with the bleeding being so heavy you thought you should speak to the GP for advice. You are hoping that the doctor will arrange an appointment for you to see your specialist as soon as you get back and sanction your plan to hold on until then. Or another option you have considered is flying home today and going to your local hospital. However, if the doctor is understanding about your work predicament but explains the seriousness of your symptoms and the need for immediate assessment, you will agree to go to the nearest emergency department today.

First words spoken to doctor – 'Hello doctor, it's Miranda Rogerson here. I'm away on business at the moment in Aberdeen and the Crohn's seems to be flaring up.'

Medical history – You were diagnosed with Crohn's disease 4 years ago. You are otherwise fit and well. Things had been fairly stable for the first 3 years until you were admitted three times in the last year for your Crohn's disease, with each admission lasting about a week and requiring steroid treatment. Since the last discharge, 4 months ago, you have been doing well. However, your specialist has said that if you have any further flare-ups, surgery may be the next option.

Drug history – You take five 25 mg tablets of azathioprine, once a day. You have no allergies.

Social history – You have a high-powered job working for a management consultancy firm in London. You stopped smoking when you were diagnosed with Crohn's disease 4 years ago. You live with your husband. You do not have any children.

Family history – Your maternal aunt has Crohn's disease. There are no other significant medical problems in your immediate family.

- Having read the information given to the simulated patient, what do you now think this station is testing?
- Make notes or discuss your thoughts with a colleague before you turn the page.

Review your approach to this station:

Tested at this station:

1. Interpersonal skills using the telephone.
2. History-taking skills.
3. Negotiating a shared management plan.

Domain 1 – Interpersonal skills

Interpersonal skills using the telephone

You need to be able to demonstrate that you are competent at conducting a consultation by telephone:

- A telephone consultation can seem relatively anonymous, so it is important to identify yourself and the patient, by name, to help build rapport.
- If there is any doubt as to the identity of the person you are speaking to, arrange to call the patient back on a number documented in their medical notes.
- One way to conceptualize how best to conduct a telephone consultation is to think about best practice in communication skills for face-to-face encounters, then accentuate these. This strategy aims to help compensate for the visual information 'lost' in such an exchange. For example:
  - Use plenty of active listening noises or words – 'uh-huh', 'yes', 'right', etc.
  - Summarize regularly.
  - Repeatedly clarify the patient's ideas, concerns and expectations so that you ensure that you address the patient's agenda.
  - Regularly 'chunk and check' – give small amounts of information, then ask the patient to clarify what has been said – as they too will not have access to visual reminders or prompts.
  - Ensure that the patient is clearly in agreement with any management plan reached.

Domain 2 – Data gathering, technical and assessment skills

History-taking skills

Without visual cues from a face-to-face consultation and the inability to conduct a physical examination, it is all the more important that you take a detailed history:

- As with a face-to-face consultation, start with open questions. What has been happening with her health recently? What has prompted her to call today? What was she hoping you could do for her?
- With telephone consultations it is useful to find out the social context in which the patient is calling. In this case she is away from home on business and feels under pressure to delay attending hospital.
- The patient is reluctant to disclose the true severity of her symptoms. Asking specific closed questions will allow you to perform an appropriate assessment:
  - How many times is she opening her bowels at the moment? How does this compare to normal?

- Are the stools well formed or loose?
- Any blood in the stools? How much? Has she had to use any pads?
- Has she vomited?
- What is her appetite like? Any weight loss recently?
- Does she feel feverish?
- Any abdominal pain? How does it compare to when she was admitted to hospital?
- Any abdominal tenderness or bloating?
- It would also be important to obtain information on her current medication and any analgesia she is taking.

Domain 3 – Clinical management skills

Negotiating a shared management plan

The patient herself knows that she should really be properly assessed in hospital but is trying to put this off for a few more days:

- Acknowledge the patient's perspective on events – she has a strong desire not to interrupt her current work commitments.
- However, make sure you clearly state the seriousness of her condition – her Crohn's appears to be flaring up and the fever, rectal bleeding and tender abdomen are all worrying signs. Does she recognize this?
- The current picture suggests a serious complication of Crohn's disease such as toxic dilatation (dangerous swelling up of her bowel), perforation of the bowel, or abscess formation. If she decides not to go to hospital today, she must realize that these are all potentially life-threatening conditions.
- If she suggests coming home today, to go to her local hospital, you should point out that even this delay could prove disastrous if she suddenly deteriorates while travelling.
- Your advice to her must be that she needs to be assessed without delay and started on appropriate treatment.
- You could suggest that if she went into hospital in Aberdeen they could easily call you and her London specialist for further information.
- Knowing all this, what does she want to do?

Knowledge base

Suggested approach to a telephone consultation

- State your name.
- Obtain the caller's name and telephone number (in case the patient has to be called back by another member of the team or the call is disconnected).
- Speak directly with the person who has a problem.
- Record the date and time of the call.
- Record the person's name, sex and age (obtain medical records if available).
- Take a detailed and structured history.

- Provide advice on treatment or disposition.
- Advise about follow-up and when to contact the doctor (for example, worsening symptoms despite treatment, symptoms failing to improve within a week, onset of new symptoms).
- Summarize the main points covered.
- Request the caller to repeat the advice given (several times throughout the consultation).
- Ask whether the person has any outstanding questions or concerns.
- Let the caller disconnect first.

From Car J, Sheikh A. Telephone consultations. *BMJ* 2003; 326: 966–969 www.bmj.com. Reproduced with permission from BMJ Publishing Group.

Take-home messages
- Telephone consultations deprive you of a wealth of visual information available from face-to-face meetings and therefore require you to take a particularly thorough history.
- If you feel unhappy agreeing to a course of action without seeing the patient, arrange for a face-to-face contact, either with yourself or with another healthcare professional.
- When agreeing a management plan with a patient on the telephone, ensure that safety-netting and follow-up are clearly understood.

Tasks

- Re-run the scenario with the patient's husband (rather than the patient) calling you seeking advice on what his wife should do.
- Re-run the scenario with the patient adamant that she will not attend hospital today. How would you manage this?
- Re-run the scenario adapting this to the local context in which you practise (e.g. if you work outside the UK).

1-minute explanations for patients

- Explain what inflammatory bowel disease is.
- Explain what inflammatory bowel disease is to a patient who does not have English as their first language.
- Explain how the medication (azathioprine) works.

Ideas for further revision

The Clinical Skills Assessment (CSA) can assess various ways of communicating with patients, such as through a third party, by telephone, or with an interpreter. Think about, and practise, how you might adapt your consultation style to meet these communication challenges.

Further reading

British Society of Gastroenterology. Guidelines for the management of inflammatory bowel disease in adults. 2011 www.bsg.org.uk

Car J, Sheikh A. Telephone consultations. *BMJ* 2003; 326: 966–969 www.bmj.com

Males, T. *Telephone Consultations in Primary Care – A practical guide.* London: Royal College of General Practitioners, 2007

NHS National Library for Health Clinical Knowledge Summaries – Crohn's disease www.cks.nhs.uk/crohns_disease

RCGP curriculum statement 15.2 – Clinical management: digestive problems www.rcgp.org.uk

Information given to candidates

Stephanie Browne is a 46-year-old woman who rarely comes to the surgery.

You note that she saw a colleague 8 years ago with acute low back pain, which settled with conservative treatment within a month.

Her only other medical history includes mild indigestion, for which she takes over-the-counter antacid medication.

Before surgery today one of the receptionists commented that Ms Browne 'can be very talkative' and joked that she didn't think Ms Browne would be in the consultation room with you for less than half an hour.

The patient enters the room walking slowly with her left hand on her lumbar spine. The first thing she says is, 'I've hurt my back and the pain has been terrible, doctor.'

- What do you think this station is testing?
- Make notes or discuss your thoughts with a colleague before you read on.

Plan your approach to this station:

Information given to simulated patient

Basic details – You are Stephanie Browne, a Caucasian 46-year-old woman who works for a small local business selling double-glazing.

Appearance and behaviour – You are naturally a talkative person and are inclined to talk at length during the consultation. You fill the silences even during any examination the doctor may perform. During the consultation you often find yourself digressing in your answers. On several occasions you will need the doctor to politely interrupt you if you are to be focused back to answering the questions they have asked.

History

Freely divulged to doctor – Two days ago you were lifting a heavy box at home in an awkward twisted position. As you started to lift you felt a sharp pain in your lower back on the left-hand side. You dropped the box. You were able to walk to the couch nearby and then lay down very carefully due to the pain. Your lower back seemed to 'seize up' and it was very painful if you tried to move.

Divulged to doctor if specifically asked – The pain is much more bearable if you lie still. You have been resting on the couch and then in bed since the injury happened. You have not had any problems passing urine or opening your bowels. You have not had any pains in your legs or any numbness or weakness. You have not felt any pins and needles in your buttocks or lower back and your sensation has been normal. Other than the pain you feel well in yourself. You have not been feverish. You have taken the occasional paracetamol for the pain but did not want to take too many tablets before seeing the doctor. Your mood is usually fine and even with this setback you are 'not too down in the dumps' about it as it got better last time and so you think the same thing should happen again.

Ideas, concerns and expectations – You were told that bed rest was the best thing for back pain when you hurt your back in a similar way 8 years ago, so you have been following this advice since the recent injury. Because the pain is not too bad if you are lying down, you believe that bringing the pain on by getting up and about must be harmful. However, if the doctor explains in a supportive and understanding manner how staying mobile is the best thing for your back, you will be responsive to this advice. You have been worrying about your cats as on a couple of occasions you felt in too much pain when trying to get up to feed them, so they went hungry. You want to know how long the problem will last and whether you should put them in the cattery.

First words spoken to doctor – 'I've hurt my back and the pain has been terrible, doctor.'

Medical history – You had a similar episode of sudden-onset lower back pain 8 years ago when you were moving house and helping your brother lift a table. However, your back has not really bothered you since that episode. You broke your left arm when you were 10 years old when you fell off a wall, but have not fractured any bones since then. You suffer from indigestion after large evening meals.

Drug history – You take Rennies® for indigestion about once a week. You are not allergic to any medication.

Social history – You work for a small local double-glazing firm in the sales office telephoning potential customers. This involves sitting at a computer for most of the day.

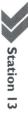

You live on your own with three cats that are much more than just pets to you. You enjoy gardening and used to walk the 1½ miles to work, although for the last 6 months you have been taking the bus. You have some good friends nearby and one younger brother who has a young family, who you get on well with. You stopped smoking 15 years ago and drink the odd glass of wine with meals.

Family history – There are no serious medical problems in your immediate family.

- Having read the information given to the simulated patient, what do you now think this station is testing?
- Make notes or discuss your thoughts with a colleague before you turn the page.

Review your approach to this station:

Tested at this station:

1. Dealing with a talkative patient.
2. Data gathering.
3. Excluding serious pathology.
4. Physical examination.
5. Management of common medical conditions presenting in primary care.

Domain 1 – Interpersonal skills

Dealing with a talkative patient

In the Clinical Skills Assessment (CSA) you have only 10 minutes for each consultation and there is often a fair amount to cover with each patient. Unless you manage talkative patients appropriately, you will run out of time and lose marks:

- In real life, many patients have a 'script' of what they want to say to the doctor, which they have rehearsed in the waiting room. Letting patients speak uninterrupted initially allows you to gather key details from the history and lets patients disclose their agenda.
- Thereafter, it is important for the doctor to take control and direct the consultation to ensure that all the main issues are covered adequately.
- Talkative patients can present a challenge to this consultation method and need to be politely, but firmly, steered back to the key points.
- One tactic is to acknowledge any digressions, then focus the patient back to the question asked, e.g. *'You are obviously worried about your cats and I can see that they are important to you, but if I can just be clear about your back pain…is the pain going down into your legs?'*
- Another tactic is to regularly summarize problems and concerns to allow you to impose some focus on the consultation.
- If you need to interrupt patients, use non-verbal as well as verbal signs, such as raising your hand, to indicate that you need to speak.
- Patients often want to continue the discussion when you are examining them. This may allow you to multitask and gain valuable additional information, although be wary of such interactions stalling the examination process.

Domain 2 – Data gathering, technical and assessment skills

Data gathering

Although the majority of acute back pain episodes resolve within a few weeks, it is important to take an adequate history to exclude serious conditions.

- History taking:
  - How did the patient sustain the injury?
  - How has she been managing since the injury?
  - Has there been any recent history of trauma?
  - Has she had back problems before?
  - Can she describe the pain – its site, nature, severity and whether it radiates?

- Does she have any pain, numbness or altered sensation in her legs?
- What makes the pain better and what makes it worse?
- Has she been taking anything for the pain?
- Does the patient suffer from osteoporosis ('thin bones')?
- Any previous fractured bones?
- Any medical history of cancer?
- Yellow flags – these represent psychosocial features associated with progression to chronic problems and disability:
  - Is the patient reluctant to do anything that brings on the pain as they think that this is harmful?
  - Does she fear the pain and is this fear making her increasingly inactive?
  - Is she more inclined to think that passive – as opposed to active – treatment will help?
  - How is her mood? Is she anxious, stressed or socially withdrawn?
  - Is there a history of problems at work?
  - Are her family overprotective?
  - An exaggerated response to examination can also be a yellow flag.

Excluding serious pathology

Red flags or indications for immediate admission must be excluded before you allow patients with acute back pain to leave the consulting room:

- Emergency action required – symptoms or signs suggestive of cauda equina syndrome or rapidly progressing neurological deficit would require immediate referral, including:
  - saddle anaesthesia
  - recent onset of bladder or bowel problems, particularly urinary retention or bowel incontinence
  - gait problems.
- Red flags – may indicate serious spinal pathology:
  - age of first presentation <20 or >50 years old
  - medical history of cancer
  - systemically unwell, e.g. fever, weight loss
  - thoracic back pain
  - pain worse if lying down
  - severe pain at night
  - intravenous drug use
  - protracted steroid use.
- If any red flags present then consider investigations including full blood count (FBC), erythrocyte sedimentation rate (ESR), urinalysis, x-ray, bone scan or referral.

Physical examination

Information from a brief, but focused, clinical examination in combination with the history helps categorize the cause of back pain:

- Any asymmetry on inspection, e.g. scoliosis?
- Where exactly is the pain? Is it definitely in the lower back rather than, say, the hips?

- Any spinal tenderness on palpation, e.g. in vertebral collapse?
- Any reduction in spinal range of movement – flexion, extension, lateral flexion and rotation?
- Assess power in legs – any weakness in knee extension, foot dorsiflexion or ankle eversion?
- Assess lower limb reflexes.
- Assess sensation – if there is a deficit, what is the distribution?
- Straight leg raises – any reduction? Unilateral or bilateral? Sciatic stretch test positive (dorsiflexion of foot increases any leg pain)?
- Do not forget to assess the patient as she walks in the consultation room and manoeuvres herself onto the examination couch.
- In the rare event of suspecting cauda equina syndrome a per rectal (PR) examination would be indicated, but this is not necessary here, and you would never be expected to perform such an examination on a simulated patient in the CSA (although you might have to do so on a model).

Domain 3 – Clinical management skills

Management of common medical conditions presenting in primary care

Appropriate advice and analgesia will aid this patient's recovery from her episode of acute simple (mechanical) lower back pain:

- General advice to help improve long-term back health, including:
  - Posture – could she improve the set-up of her chair, desk and computer at work?
  - Increased activity levels – maybe she could start walking the 1½ miles to work again rather than taking the bus?
  - Proper lifting techniques – she has injured her back twice through lifting heavy objects: does she know to bend her knees not her back?
- There are no worrying signs or symptoms and your working diagnosis should be simple (mechanical) lower back pain. Explain that the cause is probably a strain of a muscle and reassure the patient that a full recovery is likely.
- Explain that our understanding of what is best for this sort of back pain has changed and encourage her to stay mobile rather than taking to bed.
- She should aim to get back to work at the earliest opportunity to aid recovery.
- Prognosis and reassurance – you can advise her that in nine out of ten patients with this problem the pain has gone or significantly improved within 6 weeks.
- Regular analgesia, rather than PRN, such as paracetamol 1g QDS and a non-steroidal anti-inflammatory drug (NSAID) such as ibuprofen 400 mg TDS, would usually be recommended. However, this patient suffers from indigestion so you could either co-prescribe a proton pump inhibitor (PPI) (e.g. lansoprazole) with the NSAID or replace the NSAID with a weak opioid.
- Given her description of her lower back 'seizing up' you may want to consider a short course of PRN muscle relaxant, e.g. diazepam 2 mg TDS, to help ease any acute muscle spasm.

- Ask her to return in 4–6 weeks if things are not improving or sooner if she has any new symptoms or concerns.

Knowledge base

References: see Further reading below.

	Features	Management
Simple (mechanical) back pain	• Pain worse on movement • Pain worse after sitting or standing for long periods • No red flags • May be precipitating injury, e.g. lifting heavy object • Reduced range of movement of spine due to pain • Dull ache may radiate to buttocks or thighs	• Adequate analgesia: regular paracetamol and/or NSAIDs (PPI cover if >45 years old) • Encourage the patient to stay mobile and return to work, with modifications if indicated • Consider muscle relaxants, e.g. diazepam • X-rays not usually indicated

Nerve root pain	• As for simple (mechanical) back pain, but leg pain is often sharp and well localized
	• Leg pain – can be worse than any associated back pain
	• Straight leg raises reduced and stretch test positive
	• May be abnormal reflexes, e.g. absent ankle jerk, and/or altered sensation, e.g. numbness or parasthesia
		• As for simple (mechanical) back pain, plus:
		  • reassure that conservative treatment should be adequate
		  • advise may take 6–8 weeks for full recovery

Inflammatory causes of back pain	• Ankylosing spondylitis – back pain worse in morning or after inactivity • Rheumatoid arthritis (RA) – often multiple joints affected • Osteoarthritis (OA) – usually older age onset than RA	• X-rays of spine and pelvis and human leukocyte antigen (HLA) B27 antigen test for suspected ankylosing spondylitis • Rheumatoid factor, FBC and ESR if RA suspected plus referral to rheumatology and analgesia • Adequate analgesia and lifestyle advice for OA
	Features	Management
More serious causes of back pain	• Cauda equina syndrome • Aortic aneurysm • Myeloma • Vertebral collapse – secondary to osteoporosis or malignancy	• Immediate referral required for suspected cauda equina syndrome or aortic aneurysm • X-rays for suspected myeloma plus urine for Bence Jones protein and blood tests, including ESR and serum protein electrophoresis • X-rays for suspected vertebral collapse plus FBC, calcium and liver function tests (LFTs) and adequate analgesia

If simple (mechanical) back pain is not improving after 4–6 weeks, reconsider diagnosis – investigations may include FBC, alkaline phosphatase, ESR and calcium.

> **Take-home messages**
> - With talkative patients, take control of the consultation and politely, but firmly, steer them back to the key issues.
> - In back pain, be alert to red flags or any neurological findings that require immediate referral.
> - In simple (mechanical) back pain, encourage early return to normal activities, including work where appropriate, to aid recovery.

Tasks

- Re-run the scenario with the patient describing pain radiating down one of her legs into her foot. How would this change your diagnosis and the management options?
- Re-run the scenario with the patient returning to see you experiencing ongoing lower back pain 4 months after the initial injury.
- Re-run the scenario with the patient having returned from a long overseas trip to the Indian sub-continent, and with the pain being associated with night sweats and weight loss. Alternatively, if you are a MRCGP[INT] candidate, run this scenario with a patient attending with these symptoms in your own country.

1-minute explanations for patients

- Explain why it is important to keep mobile to aid recovery, even if this means feeling more pain or discomfort initially.
- Explain how the different analgesia work (paracetamol and NSAIDs).
- Explain why you don't think there is anything more serious than a simple back 'strain'.

Ideas for further revision

Time constraints in the CSA can make some stations particularly challenging. In the weeks before you take this assessment try getting your consultations down to 10 minutes to allow you to feel familiar and confident with consulting within this time frame.

Further reading

Car J, Sheikh A. 10-minute consultation: Acute low back pain. *BMJ* 2003; 327: 541 www.bmj.com

NHS Evidence Clinical Knowledge Summaries: back pain – low (without radiculopathy) www.cks.nhs.uk/back_pain_low_without_radiculopathy

NICE guidelines – Low back pain: Early management of persistent non-specific low back pain. CG88 May 2009 http://guidance.nice.org.uk/CG88/NICEGuidance/pdf/English

RCGP curriculum statement 15.9 – Clinical management: rheumatology and conditions of the musculoskeletal system (including trauma) www.rcgp.org.uk

STATION 14

Information given to candidates

Candidates note: this station is a **home visit**. You will be escorted by an invigilator to a room made to look like a patient's sitting room. The consultation will take place here.

Peter Housecliffe is a 78-year-old man who has a diagnosis of metastatic prostate cancer. The district nurse faxed the surgery with a request for a doctor to visit as shown below.

Dear Doctor

Please could you arrange an urgent visit for Peter as he is struggling with pain in his hip and is finding it difficult to mobilize.

Many thanks

DN Pearce

Peter is on the palliative care register at the practice and has been seen regularly by one of your colleagues. It is clear from reviewing the notes that his condition has been gradually deteriorating. During the last consultation his analgesia was increased with the addition of co-codamol 30/500. He is currently prescribed the following medication:

co-codamol 30/500 mg PRN (2 tablets QDS max)

As you enter the room you see a frail-looking man lying on the sofa. As he sits up to greet you he is clearly in pain. The first thing the patient says is, 'Sorry, doctor, I hope you don't mind having to let yourself in but it's a real struggle to get about at the minute.'

- What do you think this station is testing?
- Make notes or discuss your thoughts with a colleague before you read on.

Plan your approach to this station:

Information given to simulated patient

Basic details – You are Peter Housecliffe, a Caucasian 78-year-old man. You live alone.

Appearance and behaviour – You are currently lying on your sofa in the sitting room of your house. You have a bed in the same room as you have been finding it increasingly difficult to get upstairs. You are frail and feel frustrated at the loss of your independence. Movement is causing you pain in your right leg.

History

Freely divulged to doctor – You saw the district nurse this morning and she suggested it would be a good idea to contact the surgery and arrange a review as you were struggling with worsening pain in your right leg. You were planning to wait to discuss matters next week when Dr Richards would be coming for his routine visit. You know that the cancer has spread and the pain in your leg is caused by 'cancer in the bones'. This has been troubling you for a few months but has been gradually getting worse. The leg pain is worse when you move and you had been coping by taking paracetamol and using a muscle rub. Two weeks ago you were given some co-codamol tablets, too. You're most comfortable when lying in bed. You are frustrated that you are becoming more dependent on other people as you've always been able to look after yourself in the past.

Divulged to doctor if specifically asked – Over the past few days you've needed to use a stick when getting around the house due to the leg pain. It is a constant dull, gnawing ache which is mainly focused over the right hip and upper thigh, which is where the hospital doctor said the cancer was. The pain in your leg seems to be worse at night when you're trying to sleep. Your legs do not feel weak and there is no tingling or numbness. You have normal bladder control and can pass urine but have found it difficult to get to the toilet on a couple of occasions as you can't walk very quickly. You know when you need to open your bowels. Since starting the co-codamol tablets you have developed abdominal pain which is worse just before you go to the toilet. You have to strain to pass a motion and the stool is small and hard like rabbit droppings. You usually open your bowels every day without fail. Alongside the abdominal pain you also feel bloated and do not feel like eating as much as normal. You have been taking two co-codamol tablets four times a day and continue to use the muscle rub.

Ideas, concerns and expectations – You are aware that your condition is slowly deteriorating and are worried about how long you might have left to live. You think the worsening pain may be a sign that the cancer has become more aggressive. You think it may be time to get some more help at home as you're finding it harder to do the cooking and washing up. You expect the doctor to examine you and hopefully explain what's going on. You think you probably need to take stronger pain killers but worry about becoming addicted to them and that they may make you more constipated. You are particularly cautious about starting morphine as your wife died 3 days after she was prescribed morphine while in hospital with a hip fracture. You are desperate to remain in your own home as going to hospital would bring back too many memories of your wife's death. If the option of referral to the hospice is discussed you would like to know more about what the hospice can offer as the district nurse did mention they may be able to help with the pain.

First words spoken to doctor – 'Sorry, doctor, I hope you don't mind having to let yourself in but it's a real struggle to get about at the minute.'

Medical history – You were diagnosed 7 months ago with prostate cancer, which was discovered after you noticed difficulty in passing urine. The doctor at the hospital told you that the cancer had already spread to the bones at the time of diagnosis and it was in your right leg. You had TB of the lung when you were 22. You have never had any stomach ulcers or suffered from asthma.

Drug history – You take co-codamol 30/500 mg 2 tablets 4 times a day. You use a muscle rub which you buy from the local chemist.

Social history – You have lived alone since your wife died 4 years ago. You have no children. Your neighbours are helpful and do most of your shopping. You have a cleaner who comes in once a week. You prepare your own meals but are starting to find this increasingly difficult. You stopped smoking when you got married 50 years ago as your wife didn't like it. You drink the occasional glass of whisky at night.

Family history – There is no history of any relevant health problems in your family.

- Having read the information given to the simulated patient, what do you now think this station is testing?
- Make notes or discuss your thoughts with a colleague before you turn the page.

Review your approach to this station:

Tested at this station:

1. Data gathering.
2. Physical examination skills.
3. Pain control management in palliative care.
4. Coordination of care.

Domain 1 – Interpersonal skills

The initial exchanges in this scenario should reveal something about the patient's frustration regarding his loss of independence. Developing an early understanding of the patient's perspective should help frame the remainder of the consultation to ensure his autonomy is acknowledged and respected. The clinical situation is relatively simple but the exploration of the patient's ideas, concerns and expectations is very important to ensure his subsequent care can be coordinated appropriately.

Being able to quickly and effectively build rapport is a vital skill to facilitate disclosure of the patient's agenda. Some tips on how to achieve this include:

- Acknowledge the clear frustration voiced at the outset of the consultation. It is important to be observant and to comment on what you see in order to demonstrate to the patient (and examiner) that you are willing to look beyond the biological dimension. If someone appears angry or sad, then simply identifying the emotion can lead to the patient divulging further useful information.
- Direct questions can be used to ascertain what the patient is thinking and feeling at that time. Finding some phrases that feel natural for each of the ideas, concerns and expectations components can be valuable both for the Clinical Skills Assessment (CSA) and more importantly for your daily practice. If you're not sure where to begin, why not try something like *'Often people I see have been thinking about what may be behind their symptoms. Have you had any particular thoughts about what might be behind this pain?'*
- If there are no obvious issues that become apparent with your initial probing, it can be useful to ensure that you revisit this area of the consultation if you get a chance. Often patients will need to develop a sense of trust before they feel confident enough to divulge their true concerns.

Domain 2 – Data gathering, technical and assessment skills

Data gathering

Taking an accurate pain history will enable you to identify the likely cause and therefore most appropriate analgesic to use for each pain presented. SSS, OPD, RAAT can be a useful mnemonic that can be used as a template for a pain history.

By using this approach for both the hip and abdominal pain in this scenario it should be apparent that the patient is suffering from metastatic bone pain and constipation. You would then be expected to tailor your management accordingly (see Clinical management skills).

With all palliative patients it is useful to have a checklist of symptoms to cover, including:

- pain control
- breathing
- constipation
- nausea and vomiting.

These can be caused by both the cancer and the prescribed medication.

Physical examination skills

Within this scenario there would be an expectation that you would perform a focused clinical examination considering the possibility of a pathological fracture. Examination of the hip can be quickly performed using the look, feel, move approach. Lay the patient as flat as possible, then:

- Look (Inspection)
  - Any swelling, redness, deformity?
  - Any apparent leg length discrepancy?
  - Any signs that the leg is shortened and externally rotated (think hip fracture)?
- Feel (Palpation)
  - Any temperature changes?
  - Any tenderness or swelling?
- Move
  - Passive movement is usually less painful than active.
  - Assess flexion, internal and external rotation comparing both sides.
  - Special tests such as the Thomas test or Trendelenburg test can also be performed.
  - Asking the patient to walk will also allow you to assess the functional effect of their pain.

There are an increasing number of videos available online to help you develop your clinical examination skills and a well-practised examination technique is valuable for the CSA.

At this station the role-player patient will say that there is tenderness on palpation over the right hip. If you say that you wish to perform a neurological examination you will be told by the examiner to assume that this is normal. If you say that you wish to perform an abdominal examination (including rectal examination) you will be told you do not need to do this, but will be given a card with the findings: mild tenderness in the left iliac fossa, with a palpable colon, and hard stool found on rectal examination.

Domain 3 – Clinical management skills

Pain control management in palliative care

Good pain management is dependent on diagnosing the cause and type of pain present. Bone pain can be a difficult symptom to manage as it is often less responsive to opiates than other pain types. Radiotherapy, bisphosphonates, palliative surgery and nerve blocks can all be used for refractory bone pain and would be accessible through specialist palliative care services. Non-steroidal anti-inflammatory drugs (NSAIDs) can also be helpful and this is something you could offer to prescribe today.

As the patient is currently taking paracetamol in combination with a weak opiate it would be advisable to consider adding in an adjuvant, e.g. an NSAID. The World Health Organization's Pain Relief Ladder provides an effective framework on which to base analgesic prescribing (see Knowledge base). Regular pain relief is more effective than PRN. The following approach is recommended for further stepping up of analgesia, when moving to prescribing strong opioids, such as morphine:

- Continue any non-opiates currently being taken, e.g. paracetamol should be maintained.
- Calculate the initial starting dose of morphine by converting the total amount of weak opiate currently being taken. Codeine phosphate is one-tenth as potent as morphine sulphate, therefore 60 mg codeine phosphate QDS is the equivalent of 24 mg morphine sulphate over 24 hours. However, given the inadequate pain control it would be appropriate to increase this by 30–50%. Therefore a reasonable starting dose of morphine sulphate modified release (MR), taking into account tablet size, could be 20 mg BD.
- You also need to say that you would prescribe for 'breakthrough pain', such as immediate-release morphine to supplement the background analgesia, when needed (e.g. pain on movement that does not settle when resting). The breakthrough dose should be approximately one-sixth of the 24-hour background dose. What dose would this be in this scenario?
- The total amount of morphine (MR and immediate-release) taken in 24 hours on day two or three can be used to convert the immediate-release morphine to modified-release morphine sulphate to be taken every 12 hours. However, it is important to establish whether breakthrough doses are being used because the background pain remains uncontrolled (in which case increasing the MR dose is the correct action) or because background pain is well managed but movement pain is the problem. In the latter case continuing to take the existing MR and immediate-release doses, with appropriate aids and adaptations, would be most appropriate, otherwise increasing the MR dose may lead to the patient becoming drowsy.
- One of the most common side effects from opiates is constipation and it is important that this is managed proactively with appropriate laxatives. A softener laxative (docusate sodium) and a stimulant laxative (senna) in combination are usually an effective first-line treatment.
- Remember that in the CSA you are unlikely to be required to write out a full prescription within the 10 minutes, but you would be expected to demonstrate to the examiner that you know the principles, as above, of how to amend the patient's analgesia appropriately.

Coordination of care

Involving community-based palliative team members and social services in the patient's care would be appropriate at this stage. Consider discussing with the patient whether he would be happy for you to speak today to:

- a palliative care community (Macmillan) nurse
- a palliative care consultant or registrar regarding symptom management and/or hospice admission
- social services regarding care package arrangements.

Knowledge base

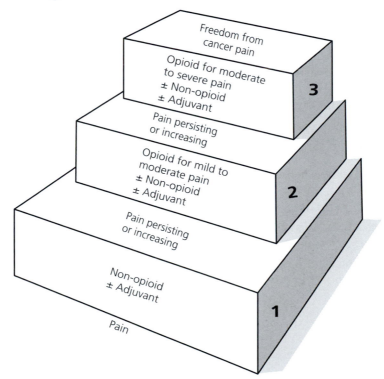

WHO pain relief ladder www.who.int/cancer/palliative/painladder/en/ (accessed 19/7/12). Reproduced with permission.

Take-home messages

- Building trust and rapport is a key skill for the CSA as it encourages patients to divulge their ideas, concerns and expectations.
- Safe and appropriate prescribing is frequently tested and the *British National Formulary (BNF)* contains a helpful section on prescribing controlled drugs.
- Referral to specialist services both in primary and secondary care can be important in the management of cancer pain.

Tasks

- Re-run the scenario with the patient having sustained a hip fracture but reluctant for hospital admission.
- Re-run the scenario with the patient needing terminal care and the district nurse consulting with you suggesting pre-emptive prescribing of end-of-life care medications.
- Re-run the scenario with the patient living with relatives who have asked for the visit. The relatives have previously insisted that they should be fully involved in any decision making regarding end-of-life care and do not want the patient to know the likely prognosis.

1-minute explanations for patients

- Describe metastatic disease.
- Explain the concept of palliative care.
- Describe the common side effects of opiates.

Ideas for further revision

Review your video consultations in order to identify phrases which work for you when trying to elicit patients' ideas, concerns and expectations. It is advisable to practise employing these in everyday surgeries to ensure that you and your patients benefit from taking a holistic approach to the 10-minute consultation.

Further reading

British Medical Association and the Royal Pharmaceutical Society of Great Britain. *British National Formulary*, 63rd edn. BMJ Publishing Group 2012

Chantal S. Pain control in palliative care. *InnovAiT* 2008; 1(4): 257–266

e-GP 16 – Physical examinations https://e-learningforhealthcare.org.uk

STATION 15

Information given to candidates

Candidates note: this station is a **telephone consultation** with a patient. Please answer the telephone when it rings. The examiner will not enter your room, but will be able to hear both you and the patient.

Jane Peterson has requested a telephone appointment regarding her daughter Katie Peterson. Katie is a 2 year old who is rarely seen at the surgery. A summary of her medical record is shown:

Katie Peterson

Age: 2 years and 2 months

8 weeks old – routine baby check: no concerns.

2 months old – vaccinations given.

3 months old – vaccinations given.

4 months old – vaccinations given.

13 months old – vaccinations given.

18 months old – viral upper respiratory tract infection.

Medications – Nil

No known drug allergies

The first thing the mother says when you pick up the phone is, 'Hello, doctor, thanks for calling back. I wanted to speak to you about my daughter Katie as she's been unwell for 3 days now.'

- What do you think this station is testing?
- Make notes or discuss your thoughts with a colleague before you read on.

Plan your approach to this station:

Information given to simulated parent

Basic details – You are Jane Peterson, a Caucasian 35-year-old mother of two. You booked a telephone consultation earlier today as you were concerned about your 2-year-old daughter Katie.

Appearance and behaviour – You are a confident but tired mother, having had little sleep over the past few days. Katie has been very clingy all day but she has just dropped off to sleep so you are somewhat relieved to have a chance to speak to the doctor in peace.

History

Freely divulged to doctor – Katie has been unwell for 3 days. She started with a runny nose and high temperature but this morning you also noticed she had developed spots on her legs and buttocks. She has been awake several times during the night for the past two nights. She has been crying on and off during the day but has settled between these episodes when she's been distracted by her favourite TV programmes. You have given her paracetamol every 6 hours and this seems to be working in bringing down her temperature.

Divulged to doctor if specifically asked – The spots are small red lumps that are visible on the legs and buttocks. The spots don't appear to be itchy and you haven't noticed any forming into blisters. Katie complained of a sore mouth yesterday and you did notice a small ulcer on the inside of her lip but didn't think much of it. Katie doesn't seem interested in food and wouldn't drink much yesterday, but she's doing better today as you're allowing her to drink through a straw. Her nappies have been wet but not as much as usual. Other than the spots, Katie's skin colour is normal. Her breathing is normal. Her lips and tongue appear moist as usual. You do not have a thermometer at home.

Ideas, concerns and expectations – You think that Katie may have chickenpox as you've seen similar spots on children through work. A friend thought it could be hand, foot and mouth disease and although you've heard of it before you don't know what causes it. Your main worry is that Katie may become dehydrated. You're also concerned about the possible dangers of being exposed to infections like chickenpox during pregnancy, although you think it's very unlikely that you'll be pregnant yet as you've only just started trying. You aren't too sure whether Katie needs to be seen face to face or whether the doctor will be able to provide advice over the telephone. You would also like to know when it will be ok for Katie to go back to nursery.

First words spoken to doctor – 'Hello, doctor, thanks for calling back. I wanted to speak to you about my daughter Katie as she's been unwell for 3 days now.'

Medical history – Katie was born at term by spontaneous vaginal delivery. There were no concerns during the pregnancy or in the first few months of her life. She was breastfed exclusively for 5 months before being weaned on to solids. She has been brought for all her vaccinations to date. You are also fit and well. You were taking the combined oral contraceptive pill but stopped 2 weeks ago as you are hoping to have another baby. You are not overweight. You're not sure whether you have had chickenpox before.

Drug history – Nil.

Social history – You are married to John and work part-time in a pre-school nursery. You have two children, Katie and her 5-year-old brother Max. Max had a cold a few weeks ago but is currently well. You have recently decided to try for another baby. You do not smoke and drink alcohol only occasionally.

Family history – There are no major health problems in your immediate family.

- Having read the information given to the simulated parent, what do you now think this station is testing?
- Make notes or discuss your thoughts with a colleague before you turn the page.

Review your approach to this station:

Tested at this station:

1. Remote assessment of the febrile child.
2. Opportunistic health promotion.
3. Using time and resources appropriately.
4. Appropriate follow-up and safety-netting.
5. Providing advice regarding common infections.

Domain 1 – Interpersonal skills

Early assessment of the expected outcome of the telephone encounter will help you to focus the consultation appropriately. Building trust and rapport can be difficult without being able to observe non-verbal cues and it is helpful to reiterate the approach to telephone consultations outlined in Station 12:

- Use plenty of active listening noises or words – 'uh-huh', 'yes', 'right', etc.
- Summarize regularly.
- Repeatedly clarify the patient's ideas, concerns and expectations so that you ensure that you address the patient's agenda.
- Regularly 'chunk and check' – give small amounts of information, then ask the patient to clarify what has been said – as they too will not have access to visual reminders or prompts.
- Ensure that the patient is clearly in agreement with any management plan reached.

Domain 2 – Data gathering, technical and assessment skills

Remote assessment of the febrile child

This is a typical telephone scenario which tests your history-taking skills in the context of remotely assessing a febrile child. The case is complicated by the challenge of seeking an accurate enough description of the rash to enable you to make a diagnosis. Both of these aspects will be facilitated by using open and closed questions:

- Assessing the febrile child can be done relatively quickly using the traffic-light approach as recommended by the National Institute for Health and Clinical Excellence (NICE) (see Knowledge base). Asking specific closed questions about skin colour, activity, respiratory function, hydration status and checking for red-flag signs of meningism will allow you to gather much of the necessary information to decide whether a child needs to be seen face to face.
- Asking the carer to describe the rash in as much detail as possible is helpful. Try to avoid settling on a diagnosis too early in the consultation. If someone says a rash looks like chickenpox it is important to still ask for a description of the exact appearance.
- It is useful to explore the mother's ideas, concerns and expectations early in a consultation of this type as it will allow you to frame the consultation appropriately.

Opportunistic health promotion

By exploring the mother's concerns it should become apparent that she is trying for another baby. Pre-conception advice can be offered but it may be helpful to signpost this during the consultation, revisiting it later so as not to interfere with the flow of data gathering.

Domain 3 – Clinical management skills

Using time and resources appropriately

A main focus of this scenario is to test your ability to use clinical time and resources appropriately. An accurate history should allow you to make a diagnosis of hand, foot and mouth disease and to ascertain that Katie is coping reasonably well with the infection. One question that needs to be considered is whether you need to assess the child face to face or whether you are confident enough from the information available to provide telephone advice. Telephone advice can be convenient to both patients and doctors, but you need to bear in mind the potential increased risk of misdiagnosis. It is advisable to always ask yourself whether telephone advice is appropriate in a given situation and to review this throughout the consultation. There are several factors which will influence the answer to this question:

● working and differential diagnoses
● the severity of the presentation
● the preference of the patient or carer
● any relevant medical history.

Appropriate follow-up and safety-netting

You would generally be expected to be able to make a diagnosis and offer appropriate reassurance over the telephone in this situation, but patient safety is obviously paramount, so if you are concerned that a patient needs to be seen face to face, this should be arranged promptly. Appropriate safety-netting involves giving clear information regarding the expected course of illness, specific signs which would suggest deterioration, and what to do should this occur. In this instance:

● Hand, foot and mouth disease is usually a mild self-limiting infection which generally improves within a week or so. The risk of dehydration is the biggest concern as mouth ulcers often make children reluctant to drink.
● Dehydration is often difficult to assess. Irritability, dry lips/tongue and decreased urine output are signs to look out for, but encouraging the carer to use their instinct can also help. If they are concerned that their child is not drinking enough, contact with a health professional is advisable.
● It is useful to provide information about who to contact both in and out of hours.

Providing advice regarding common infections

It is important to provide accurate information about nursery and school absence and measures that can be taken to avoid spread of infectious diseases:

- Frequent hand-washing is an effective measure and this should be continued for several weeks, particularly after nappies are changed as the virus can continue to be excreted in the stool after the acute infection has resolved.
- School avoidance is not recommended for hand, foot and mouth disease as the infection is generally mild, with a low risk of further complications. Patients with chickenpox should be advised to wait 5 days from the onset of the rash before they return to a school environment.
- It is important that a pregnant woman who comes into contact with someone who has a potentially infectious rash remains vigilant and speaks to their midwife or GP. Chickenpox, rubella, measles and parvovirus B19 (slapped-cheek disease) can all complicate pregnancy in non-immune individuals. Promptly checking antibody levels helps guide any necessary treatment. See *BMJ* article in Further reading.

Knowledge base

The traffic-light approach to assessing children with a feverish illness provides a framework for deciding whether care can be safely provided at home or whether

	Green – low risk	Amber – intermediate risk	Red – high risk
Colour	• Normal colour of skin, lips and tongue	• Pallor reported by parent/career	• Pale/mottled/ashen/blue
Activity	• Responds normally to social cues • Content/smiles • Stays awake or awakens quickly • Strong normal cry/ not crying	• Not responding normally to social cues • Wakes only with prolonged stimulation • Decreased activity • No smile	• No response to social cues • Appears ill to a healthcare professional • Unable to rouse or if roused does not stay awake • Weak, high-pitched or continuous cry
Respiratory		• Nasal flaring • Tachypnoea: – RR >50 breaths/minute age 6–12 months – RR >40 breaths/minute age >12 months • Oxygen saturation ≤95% in air • Crackles	• Grunting • Tachypnoea: – RR >60 breaths/minute • Moderate or severe chest indrawing
Hydration	• Normal skin and eyes • Moist mucous membranes	• Dry mucous membrane • Poor feeding in infants • CRT ≥3 seconds • Reduced urine output	• Reduced skin turgor
Other	• None of the amber or red symptoms or signs	• Fever for ≥5 days • Swelling of a limb or joint • Non-weight bearing/ not using an extremity • A new lump >2 cm	• Age 0–3 months, temperature ≥38°C • Age 3–6 months, temperature ≥39°C • Non-blanching rash • Bulging fontanelle • Neck stiffness • Status epilepticus • Focal neurological signs • Focal seizures • Bile-stained vomiting

CRT: capillary refill time
RR: respiratory rate

further assessment is required. If all green features are present with no amber or red, the child can usually be managed at home. If any amber features are present, assessment in a face-to-face setting is advised. Red features should trigger an urgent assessment (within 2 hours).

From: NICE guidelines – Feverish illness in children: Assessment and initial management in children younger than 5 years. Clinical Guidelines 47. May 2007 www.nice.org.uk/CG047. Reproduced with permission.

> **Take-home messages**
> * The remote assessment of a child with a feverish illness needs to have a clear structure to ensure the information required to make an accurate assessment is elicited.
> * Appropriate safety-netting involves providing clear instruction as to what to expect and how to respond if the clinical condition fails to follow the expected course.
> * Opportunistic health promotion can and should be provided where possible.

Tasks

* Re-run the scenario with the patient needing face-to-face assessment but with the mother unable to bring her to the surgery as she has no available transport.
* Re-run the scenario with the mother 14 weeks pregnant and concerned about the possibility of exposure to chickenpox.
* Re-run the scenario with the mother concerned about the risk of febrile convulsions given that her son had a fit when he was unwell with chickenpox at a similar age.

1-minute explanations for patients

* Explain the diagnosis of hand, foot and mouth disease.
* Explain a febrile convulsion.
* Explain the importance of folic acid in pregnancy.

Ideas for further revision

Reflect on your skills at remotely assessing both children and adults. Discuss with your peers and colleagues their thresholds for face-to-face assessment.

Further reading

Health Protection Agency. Guidance on infection control in schools and other childcare settings www.hpa.org.uk

MacMahon E. Investigating the pregnant woman exposed to a child with a rash. *BMJ* 2012; 344: e1790

Neighbour R. *The Inner Consultation: How to develop an effective and intuitive consulting style*. 2nd edn. Radcliffe Medical Press. 2004

NICE guidelines – Feverish illness in children: Assessment and initial management in children younger than 5 years. Clinical Guidelines 47. May 2007 www.nice.org.uk/CG047

Information given to candidates

Sara Reddy is a 32-year-old patient.

6/12 ago – fractured maxilla

8/12 ago - headache

9/12 ago - tired all the time

18/12 ago – depression

Drug history:

Citalopram 20 mg OD

Microgynon 30

A pop-up box on the computer records reminds you that a routine contraceptive pill check is overdue.

The first thing the patient says as she enters the consultation room is, 'Hi. The doctor at the hospital said to see you if I needed more pain killers. I've run out of the ones they gave me.'

- What do you think this station is testing?
- Make notes or discuss your thoughts with a colleague before you read on.

Plan your approach to this station:

Information given to simulated patient

Basic details – You are Sara Reddy, a 32-year-old receptionist for a large insurance company. You have been married to Steve for 5 years and have no children.

Appearance and behaviour – You are casually dressed in a long-sleeved jumper. You come across as anxious to get a prescription and do not wish to spend long talking. You are not keen to be examined and if asked to roll up your sleeve/take off your jumper for a blood pressure (BP) check you are reluctant as you are trying to conceal large bruises on your arms.

History

Freely divulged to doctor – You attended the emergency department 2 weeks ago and were found to have a fractured clavicle. You have been taking co-codamol 2 tablets four times a day and wearing a sling most days. The pain is getting better but you still feel it on and off throughout the day and could do with some more pain killers, particularly as it's been worse since you ran out a few days ago.

Divulged to doctor if specifically asked – You are reluctant to divulge the details of how you fractured your clavicle and try to change the subject, simply mentioning you had 'a bit of a fall'. If asked about how you fractured your cheekbone 6 months ago you are initially reluctant to give details and state that you 'tripped down the stairs at home'. If the doctor enquires as to whether anyone else has been involved in these incidents you become quiet and have to work hard not to cry. After a period of silence, and if you feel that the doctor is someone you can trust, you admit your husband Steve has hit you on several occasions in the past and pushed you down the stairs 2 weeks ago following an argument about you going out with some friends. He seems to be angry all the time and is very controlling of who you spend time with. His anger has worsened in recent months and you're scared about what might happen now. He threatened to kill you last week if you ever told anyone about him hitting you, but he's never said that before and was drunk at the time. You don't think he even remembers anything about that night. Your fractured cheekbone occurred when Steve pushed you and you fell onto a coffee table.

Ideas, concerns and expectations – You don't know what to do but you're scared for your safety. You think Steve will come after you even if you try to leave him and you are initially desperate that nobody else be told about what you have disclosed. You expect confidentiality and refuse to give permission for the doctor to contact 'the authorities'. You know deep down that you have to get out of the relationship but you need some time to work out how. You don't think you're in any immediate danger as Steve is working away for the next week. You would be happy to talk to someone about what your options are for dealing with the situation and possibly finding a house of your own away from Steve.

First words spoken to doctor – 'Hi. The doctor at the hospital said to see you if I needed more pain killers. I've run out of the ones they gave me.'

Medical history – Depression. Fractured maxilla 6/12 ago.

Drug history – You have been taking co-codamol 2 tablets up to four times a day for the past 2 weeks. You have been taking citalopram 20 mg once a day for depression for the last 18 months. You also take the combined contraceptive pill, Microgynon 30. You have no known drug allergies.

Social history – You have been living with Steve for 8 years after meeting through a friend at work. He first hit you when drunk 4 years ago but had not done so again until 6 months ago. You smoke around 10 cigarettes a day and drink alcohol occasionally when you go out with friends. Your mum lives in Scotland and would be happy for you to go and stay with her there.

Family history – There are no serious medical problems in your immediate family. Your dad died in a motorbike accident when you were young.

- Having read the information given to the simulated patient, what do you now think this station is testing?
- Make notes or discuss your thoughts with a colleague before you turn the page.

Review your approach to this station:

Tested at this station:

1. Recognizing the possibility of domestic abuse.
2. Responding to a disclosure of domestic abuse.
3. Reaching a shared management plan.

Domain I – Interpersonal skills

Recognizing the possibility of domestic abuse

Domestic abuse is an under-recognized yet major public health problem which has long-term health consequences for those it affects. Twenty five per cent of women will experience domestic violence and the fact that it is a clinical priority for the RCGP (2011–2013) demonstrates the need for trainees to be aware of their roles and responsibilities in this area. Many victims of domestic abuse find their relationships with friends and family controlled to the extent that the GP may be one of the few people they can turn to for support and advice. How GPs recognize the possibility and respond to a disclosure of domestic abuse is therefore vital.

- It is important to be aware of the possibility that domestic abuse can affect people from any and every background. Physical injuries, recurrent gynaecological problems, substance misuse and mental health problems are more prevalent in victims of domestic abuse and should be a trigger for clinicians to consider sensitively asking whether abuse may be taking place.
- It is vital that care is taken when trying to ascertain whether domestic abuse has taken/is taking place. Asking when a partner is present or waiting outside may place the victim in increased danger.
- Pre-planned statements can be a helpful way of opening the door for a victim to divulge information, e.g. 'I have seen some people with injuries such as these which have occurred as a result of someone hurting them. Do you ever feel in danger at home?'

Responding to a disclosure of domestic abuse

Responding to a disclosure appropriately is the second skill tested in this scenario. Five key messages can be given which provide a platform for a victim to get the support they need:

- 'Thank you for telling me' – many victims feel a sense of guilt for betraying the trust of their abuser and may question whether they have done the right thing.
- 'I believe you' – often over time an individual's self-esteem will have diminished to the extent that they think they have no voice of their own.
- 'It's not your fault' – many victims have been led to believe that they deserve to be abused for failing to provide for their partners. Arguments about household chores are frequently a stimulus for abuse.
- 'You have the right to be safe at home' – it is a basic human right for everyone to feel safe.
- 'There is support available' – often it will be impossible for a GP to provide the care and support needed for the victim, but facilitating access to specialist services is usually appropriate.

Domain 2 – Data gathering, technical and assessment skills

Responding to a disclosure of domestic abuse (continued)

Following disclosure it is important for a clinician to assess the risks posed to an individual and any children who may be exposed to ongoing domestic abuse. The formal CAADA–DASH Risk Identification Checklist can be used following disclosure (see Further reading), but within the history there is also the opportunity to explore specific points which may help identify those at risk of serious harm. The C-SPECSS acronym is a helpful reminder of some of these:

- Children – the presence of children within an abusive relationship necessitates consideration of their social and physical well-being. The safety of children in this setting would be a priority issue.
- Separation – it is known that victims trying to leave an abusive relationship are at increased risk of serious violence. Issues over child custody are also frequent triggers for abuse.
- Pregnancy – violence often begins or increases during pregnancy and even more so after a baby is born.
- Escalation – it is important to gather information as to whether violence has been increasing over a period of time. Those experiencing escalating violence are clearly at heightened risk of life-threatening harm.
- Cultural issues – honour-based violence is increasingly recognized as a source of serious abuse, with a risk of victims being murdered. No race or culture condones violence within marriage or between partners and their children. Some minority groups, however, face barriers which can deter or prevent them from reporting such incidents.
- Stalking – high-risk victims of domestic abuse may also be subject to stalking related to controlling behaviours.
- Sexual abuse – victims of sexual assault are frequently subject to more serious injury.

Domain 3 – Clinical management skills

Reaching a shared management plan

Helping a patient decide what to do following a disclosure of domestic abuse tests your ability to reach a shared management plan. It is important to avoid being directive and instead to walk them through the options. It can be useful to enquire as to what the patient wants you to do as a starting point for these discussions.

- Be aware that for a variety of reasons some people may make a decision that seems irrational. A real fear of escalating violence or an ongoing desire for a relationship to continue can be a barrier to change.
- Never offer to act as an intermediary between your patient and the perpetrator as this can expose both you and them to danger.
- Develop awareness of support services, both locally and nationally. Helplines, domestic violence support agencies and the police are all potential access points for further help.

- Encourage the victim to make a safety plan (see Knowledge base).
- It is also important to ensure that any health needs are met which in this scenario would involve prescribing appropriate analgesia.

Knowledge base

Safety planning can cover various stages and should be facilitated by whomever domestic abuse is disclosed to when there is ongoing risk of further harm. The Department of Health resource recommends covering the following areas:

Safety in the relationship

- Places to avoid when abuse starts (such as the kitchen, where there are many potential weapons).
- People a woman can turn to for help or let know that they are in danger.
- Asking neighbours or friends to call 999 if they hear anything to suggest a woman or her children are in danger.
- Places to hide important phone numbers, such as helpline numbers.
- How to keep the children safe when abuse starts.
- Teaching the children to find safety or get help, perhaps by dialling 999.
- Keeping important personal documents in one place so that they can be taken if a woman needs to leave suddenly.
- Letting someone know about the abuse so that it can be recorded (important for cases that go to court or immigration applications, for example).

Leaving in an emergency

- Packing an emergency bag and hiding it in a safe place in case a woman needs to leave in an emergency.
- Plans for who to call and where to go (such as a domestic violence refuge).
- Things to remember to take: documents, medication, keys or a photo of the abuser (useful for serving court documents).
- Access to a phone.
- Access to money or credit/debit cards that a woman has perhaps put aside.
- Plans for transport.
- Plans for taking clothes, toiletries and toys for the children.
- Taking any proof of the abuse, such as photos, notes or details of people who know about it.

Helplines

National agencies can help support victims to find safe emergency refuge accommodation and put them in touch with people who can ensure that they're protected. This can be done without them having to tell them their name. The helplines include:

- English National Domestic Violence Helpline: 0808 2000 247
- Men's Advice Line: 0808 801 0327
- Wales Domestic Abuse Helpline: 0808 80 10 800
- Dyn Wales/Dyn Cymru (for men in Wales): 0808 801 0321

- Scottish Domestic Abuse Helpline: 0800 027 1234
- Northern Ireland Women's Aid 24-hour Domestic Violence Helpline: 0800 917 1414
- Broken Rainbow Helpline (for lesbian, gay, bisexual and transgender people): 0300 999 5428
- Respect Phoneline (for people who are abusive to partners and want help to stop): 0808 802 4040
- Forced Marriage Unit: 020 7088 0151.

Confidentiality issues

Danger of immediate serious harm to the victim and the impact of domestic abuse on children can often require information sharing with agencies such as multi-agency risk assessment conferences, safeguarding children teams or the police. Consent to share information is always preferable, but there may be instances where this consent is withheld. The Department of Health's *Responding to Domestic Abuse* handbook (see Further reading) offers guidance on what can be done in this relatively rare situation:

- Always seek a woman's permission to share information.
- Given current legislation in England (section 115 of the Crime and Disorder Act 1998) it is permissible to pass information without permission to another agency in situations where:
  - the courts request information about a specific case, or
  - there is significant risk of harm to the woman, her children or somebody else if information is not passed on.
- If you do pass on information without permission, you should be completely sure that your decision does not place somebody at risk of greater violence. You will need to be able to justify your decision. Medical defence organizations and local safeguarding teams can offer information on what disclosure may be justified.

Take-home messages

- Domestic abuse is under-recognized.
- GPs have a key role in identifying domestic abuse and supporting patients to make informed choices.
- Confidentiality can be broken in certain circumstances, e.g. if children are involved.

Tasks

- Re-run the scenario with the patient being a male victim of intimate partner violence.
- Re-run the scenario with the patient being the perpetrator of such violence, seeking anger management.
- Re-run the scenario with there being young children at home with an immediate threat requiring prompt intervention.

1-minute explanations for patients

- Explain what is meant by a safety plan.
- Describe circumstances surrounding domestic abuse when confidentiality may need to be broken.
- Describe your local child safeguarding procedures.

Ideas for further revision

Responding effectively to a disclosure of domestic abuse is dependent on having the necessary knowledge and skills to offer support to the victim. Review your practice policy/information regarding disclosure of domestic abuse and read your local safeguarding children board's guidance on the issue.

Further reading

CAADA frequently asked questions about Multi-Agency Risk Assessment Conferences (MARACs) available from: www.caada.org.uk/aboutus/Key%20 CAADA%20FAQs%20-%20MARACs.pdf

CAADA-DASH Risk Identification Checklist available from: www.caada.org.uk/ dvservices/RIC_and_severity_of_abuse_grid_and_IDVA_practice_guidance.pdf

Department of Health. *Responding to Domestic Abuse: A handbook for health professionals.* London: Department of Health, 2005. Available from: www.dh.gov. uk/prod_consum_dh/groups/dh_digitalassets/@dh/@en/documents/digitalasset/ dh_4126619.pdf [Accessed April 2012]

eGP Module 10_1a_13 Domestic violence available from: http://e-lfh.org.uk/ projects/egp/index.html

RCGP curriculum statement 10.1 – Women's health www.rcgp-curriculum.org.uk/ PDF/curr_10_1_Womens_Health.pdf

Schroeder K. Assessing domestic abuse in women. *InnovAiT* 2011; 4(7): 420–421

STATION 17

Information given to candidates

George Agnew is a 72-year-old patient who lives with his long-term partner, Hilary.

George has asked for an appointment to talk about his concerns regarding Hilary's health.

George is attending on his own today.

As George enters the consulting room he says, 'I'm concerned that Hilary's memory seems to be going. I think it might be the beginnings of Alzheimer's. After 30 years together I'm worried our relationship is breaking down.'

- What do you think this station is testing?
- Make notes or discuss your thoughts with a colleague before you read on.

Plan your approach to this station:

Information given to simulated carer

Basic details – You are George Agnew, a Caucasian 72-year-old retired schoolteacher. You have come to the surgery to discuss your concerns regarding the health of your long-term male partner, Hilary Mendle, who is 68 years old.

Appearance and behaviour – You are well presented, wearing a jacket and tie. You are a little anxious as you believe that seeing the doctor today will probably set in train a series of events that will take matters partly out of your hands. In some sense, you are relieved at this, having been carrying around for some time now your own 'secret' – namely, your fear that Hilary is showing signs of Alzheimer's.

History

Freely divulged to doctor – Hilary's memory started to get worse about a year ago. There has been a gradual decline over that time. Now he needs to write lists to remind himself about even the smallest things. More recently he has been forgetting the way home from the local shops and on two occasions you went out to find him wandering nearby. He used to be a keen letter writer but now finds it difficult to write even a short postcard. He gets confused in new surroundings. Your friends have started to comment.

Divulged to doctor if specifically asked – He has never been an aggressive man, but last week Hilary became agitated and upset at home after you had rearranged the furniture in the front room, and he smashed one of your treasured school photos. You were shocked when he did not recognize some old friends of you both when you bumped into them in the supermarket. Hilary has been well in himself otherwise – no chesty coughs or complaints of any pains. He has never smoked. Hilary does seem to recognize the problems he is having with his memory, but he dismisses it as 'just old age'. He got quite angry when you suggested coming to see the doctor today as he denied that anything was wrong. Hilary does not drive. You are now having to do most of the household chores yourself.

Ideas, concerns and expectations – You have been putting off coming to see the doctor for several months as you did not want to accept what was happening. You have been together for more than 30 years and feel that you would not know how to cope if, as you fear, a diagnosis of Alzheimer's disease is made. Both of you have always been very private people and the idea of having to explain your domestic situation to 'strangers' from numerous agencies who might be involved in Hilary's care is something you worry about greatly. The recent aggressive episodes really concerned you and prompted you to attend today. You want to know whether there is anything that can be done to help with these in particular. You suspect that the doctor will talk about Hilary having to go into a residential home, but you want him to stay at home as long as he can. You want to know how long it will be before he stops recognizing you. You have heard about medication that can help and want to ask the doctor about this.

First words spoken to doctor – 'I'm concerned that Hilary's memory seems to be going. I think it might be the beginnings of Alzheimer's. After 30 years together I'm worried our relationship is breaking down.'

Medical history – You are in good physical health. Hilary has been a fit and active man all his life and apart from a hip replacement 2 years ago has been 'in rude health'.

Drug history – Hilary takes the odd pain killer for arthritis but does not have any regular medication.

Social history – You both worked as teachers in private schools until you both retired 7 years ago. You met Hilary 30 years ago at a teaching conference and have been living together since then. Your respective families never enquired in too much detail about your relationship and over time you have both lost touch with them. You were both active in your retirement, travelling abroad and playing bridge for the local club.

Family history – As far as you are aware, there are no major health problems in Hilary's family.

- Having read the information given to the simulated carer, what do you now think this station is testing?
- Make notes or discuss your thoughts with a colleague before you turn the page.

Review your approach to this station:

Tested at this station:

1. Understanding of equality and diversity issues.
2. Taking a history from a third party.
3. Supporting a patient's carer.

Domain 1 – Interpersonal skills

Understanding of equality and diversity issues

The GP curriculum states that promoting equality and valuing diversity are at the heart of the curriculum, and that diversity is about recognizing and valuing difference in its broadest sense. The carer in this scenario happens to be in a same-sex relationship. You need to avoid being judgemental or making assumptions that could lead to a breakdown of trust within the consultation:

- When patients, relatives or carers use gender-neutral terms such as 'partner', be alert to the fact that they could be referring to a same-sex partner.
- Do not make assumptions regarding the sexual orientation of a patient, carer or relative. If you get it wrong (e.g. by asking about a male patient's 'wife' or 'girlfriend' when his partner is male), some patients may decide not to correct you but will feel that you are not a doctor who could be responsive to their needs and may simply book again to see someone else.
- If you do get it wrong and are corrected by the patient, carer or relative, although you may be embarrassed at your error it is best just to apologize for your mistake and move on.
- You may have strong personal beliefs around sexuality issues, but in your role as a medical practitioner you need to be non-judgemental and remain professional.
- In *Good Medical Practice*, the General Medical Council makes clear that the duties of a doctor include never discriminating unfairly against patients or colleagues by allowing personal views on issues such as sexual orientation to adversely affect professional relationships with them (paragraph 7 – see Further reading).
- In this scenario, being accepting and understanding of the worries George has regarding potentially having to disclose his and Hilary's domestic situation to numerous outside agencies – to 'strangers' – is a key skill that will allow you to demonstrate your awareness of equality and diversity issues to the examiner.

Domain 2 – Data gathering, technical and assessment skills

Taking a history from a third party

In many circumstances taking a history from someone who is not the patient can be problematical, but when the presenting complaint is memory difficulties and aggressive behaviour it is essential to have a clear history from a third party:

- When did George first notice problems with Hilary's memory? Can he give examples? How have things progressed? Has anyone else commented on this?
- Have the changes been gradual or stepwise?

- Has Hilary's personality changed in any way?
- Hilary was aggressive last week and this was out of character for him. When and where did this episode occur, e.g. was it at dusk? Were there any obvious triggers? Has Hilary been unwell over the last week, e.g. with a chesty cough or going to the toilet more frequently to urinate?
- Has Hilary been complaining of any other problems – any pains, weight loss or low mood?
- Have there been any episodes where Hilary has put himself – or others – in danger, e.g. leaving the gas on?
- Does Hilary suffer from any other medical conditions, such as diabetes or high blood pressure?
- Does he take any medication? Has he started any new medicines over the last year?
- Has Hilary ever had a heart attack or stroke?
- Does he smoke?
- Does he drive?
- What does Hilary think about what has been happening? Does he recognize that there is a problem?
- Is there a reason why George has come to the surgery on his own? Does Hilary know that George is here today?

Domain 3 – Clinical management skills

Supporting a patient's carer

George has come to you today to seek help and support regarding his concerns about Hilary. You need to provide genuine support to George as a carer by acknowledging his worries, exploring his feelings about the situation and providing information on what will happen next:

- Thank George for coming to see you today and explain how the information he is able to give about Hilary is extremely useful.
- Empathize that it must have been very difficult to carry on for so long without discussing his concerns with anyone else.
- George is fairly convinced that Hilary has Alzheimer's disease. Why does he think this? Has he had previous experience of people with dementia?
- What are George's thoughts about what will happen next? Does he have any specific worries or concerns?
- Hilary does seem to have some idea that his memory is worsening, but he dismisses it as 'just old age'. What does George think about this? Might Hilary be using denial as a coping strategy?
- Explain that there could be a number of different causes of Hilary's symptoms (e.g. depression, the effect of medication, or other medical problems such as hormone or vitamin deficiencies) and that a diagnosis would be made only after a proper assessment.
- Hilary refused to come to the surgery today, but would he accept a home visit? If Hilary is adamant that he will not see a doctor, you would need to explain to George how it is difficult for you to go against Hilary's expressed wishes (see Knowledge base).

- Explain that if Hilary allows you to visit you will do some simple memory tests and may need to take blood to exclude various physical causes. If appropriate, you may end up referring him to the memory clinic for further specialist assessment.
- Advise George that Hilary will be involved in all stages of the investigation process. Explain how you would ask Hilary how much he wanted to know about his problem, and would never force information on him against his wishes.
- Advise George that if a diagnosis of dementia is subsequently made, there are support services available for carers, including:
  - provision of home-care packages to support patients in their own home
  - psychological therapies available for carers
  - carer support groups and carer training programmes
  - respite care
  - input from district nurses to give advice about nursing care
  - support from community psychiatric nurses
  - Age UK, the UK's largest organization working with and for older people, has local support groups and a useful website aimed at carers, too (see Further reading).
- George is particularly worried about the recent aggressiveness. Explain that there may be a number of reasons for this, e.g. an infection or the recent change to a familiar environment that has upset him. Say that you can assess this when you visit, but that there are therapies available to deal with such challenging behaviour (see Knowledge base). Advise George not to make any changes about the house or to their routines at the moment.

Knowledge base – Dementia

References: see Further reading below

Definition	• A global impairment of cognitive function without clouding of consciousness
Living with dementia	• One in twenty aged >65 years • One in five aged >80 years
Types	• Alzheimer's disease – most common form (approximately 60%) • Vascular dementia – progression may be stepwise (approximately 20%) • Lewy body dementia – can have hallucinations and parkinsonism • Frontotemporal lobe dementia – rare, includes Pick's disease, often affects those <65 years old. Memory may be intact but personality can change
Investigations	• Appropriate history and examination to exclude other causes, e.g. depression, medication, or other medical conditions • Mini-Mental State Examination – 30-point formal cognitive test or abbreviated tools, such as the Abbreviated Mental Test Score • Blood tests – full blood count (FBC), urea and electrolytes (U&E), thyroid function tests (TFTs), glucose, liver function tests (LFTs), calcium, vitamin B12 and folate • Midstream specimen urine test if delirium is a possibility • Chest x-ray or electrocardiogram (ECG) as determined by clinical presentation • National Institute for Health and Clinical Excellence (NICE) recommend not routinely testing for syphilis or HIV unless indicated

(continued)

Referral	• To specialist memory clinics for further assessment of cognitive, behavioural and global functioning by elderly care psychiatry teams. Imaging may subsequently be arranged, e.g. magnetic resonance imaging (MRI)
Interventions	• Acetylcholinesterase inhibitors (e.g. donepezil, galantamine, rivastigmine) may be considered for mild to moderate Alzheimer's disease • Review and treat vascular risk factors • Care plans to maximize independent activity and help support carers • Reality orientation – regularly orientating people in time, place and key facts • For challenging behaviour – address environmental and psychosocial factors. National Institute for Health and Clinical Excellence (NICE) list non-pharmacological interventions, including: aromatherapy, animal-assisted therapy, massage, music and dance therapy, multisensory stimulation

Mental Capacity Act 2005 for England and Wales	• Came into force in April 2007
	• A statutory framework to empower and protect those who may lack capacity to make decisions for themselves
	• Adults presumed to have capacity unless proven otherwise
	• Individuals must be given all practicable support before it is concluded that they are not able to make their own decisions
	• Individuals are able to make what might be seen as an unwise decision
	• Anything done for or on behalf of individuals without capacity:
	  • must be in their best interests
	  • should restrict their rights and basic freedoms as little as possible
	• Lasting powers of attorney – individuals can appoint someone to make health and welfare decisions on their behalf if they lose capacity at some future time

---

Take-home messages

• Avoid making assumptions about people's sexual orientation.

• Only in exceptional circumstances should you go against the express wishes of patients.

• Thorough assessment is required of anyone presenting with cognitive impairment.

• Supporting carers is a key role of the primary healthcare team.

Tasks

● Re-run the scenario as a subsequent home visit to see Hilary. What would you say if he asks you why you are there? How would you sensitively start to explore Hilary's memory problems?

● Re-run the scenario with Hilary presenting as a widower living on his own and concerned about his memory. How might this change your management?

● Re-run the scenario with Hilary's partner George consulting with you as things have reached crisis point, with Hilary becoming aggressive and wandering outside most nights.

● You may be unfamiliar, if a non-UK candidate, with handling the issue of same-sex partners. If you are working in the UK, we suggest you make sure that you are familiar with, and practise using, gender-neutral terms. MRCGP[INT] candidates should adjust the scenario to their own cultural support systems, e.g. you may want to have a daughter worried about her father who is living with them.

1-minute explanations for patients

- Explain to a patient what dementia is.
- Explain to a carer what dementia is.
- Explain to a patient what further assessments will take place to help reach a diagnosis regarding memory problems.

Ideas for further revision

Your local mental health unit should have a memory clinic, probably run by the elderly care psychiatry team. Arrange to spend some time with them sitting in on clinics and speaking to members of the multidisciplinary team. Find out what they expect of primary care before referring patients with suspected dementia to specialist services.

Further reading

Age UK www.ageuk.org.uk

Alzheimer's Society www.alzheimers.org.uk

Breen DA, Breen DP, Moore JW, Breen PA, O'Neill D. Driving and dementia. *BMJ* 2007; 334: 1365–1369 www.bmj.com

General Medical Council *Good Medical Practice.* London, 2006 www.gmc-uk.org/static/documents/content/GMP_0910.pdf

Mental Capacity Act 2005 www.justice.gov.uk/guidance/protecting-the-vulnerable/mental-capacity-act/index.htm

NICE guidelines 42 – Dementia: Supporting people with dementia and their carers in health and social care. Quick reference guide. March 2011 http://guidance.nice.org.uk/cg42/quickrefguide/pdf/english

RCGP curriculum statement 3.4 – Promoting equality and valuing diversity; RCGP curriculum statement 9 – Care of older adults www.rcgp.org.uk

Information given to candidates

> Sarah Chatwich is a 42-year-old patient who rarely comes to the surgery. Previous entries in her records are for smears and minor illnesses.
>
> A pop-up box on her computer records reminds you that she has impaired hearing and lip reads.

As the patient enters the room she says, 'I've been feeling so tired and run down recently, doctor – I'm worried there's something seriously wrong.'

- What do you think this station is testing?
- Make notes or discuss your thoughts with a colleague before you read on.

Plan your approach to this station:

Information given to simulated patient

Basic details – You are Sarah Chatwich, a Caucasian 42-year-old single woman who works full-time as a manager in an computer firm.

Appearance and behaviour – You are well presented. You wear hearing aids in both ears. You have minimal hearing and understand people primarily by lip reading. Consequently, you need to have a clear view of the doctor's face. You will miss what is being said unless the doctor speaks slowly and clearly, and faces you when speaking. You get annoyed if people patronize you because of your hearing impairment and you will challenge the doctor if you feel that his or her behaviour is inappropriate in this regard.

History

Freely divulged to doctor – You have been feeling run down for several months now. You are tired all the time and lack energy. When you were on holiday in the USA recently your American friend said that you might have a hormone problem and that you should see your doctor when you got home. You are putting on weight – about a stone over the last year – despite trying to eat a healthy diet. When in America, even though the weather was fairly warm, you found yourself wearing more layers than the rest of your group, and looking back you have been feeling the cold more for a while.

Divulged to doctor if specifically asked – Your periods are regular but have been getting heavier over recent months. You get constipated – something you never used to suffer from – with hard stools, and you are now opening your bowels only twice a week (last year you used to go almost every day). You feel as though you have been slowed down over the last 3 or 4 months, and you sometimes find it difficult to concentrate on things, but you put this down to being so tired. You have not felt depressed. You have no problems sleeping or with your appetite. You are not going to the toilet to urinate more frequently and you are not excessively thirsty. You have never suffered from chest pain or had any heart problems. You have never suffered from high blood pressure or headaches.

Ideas, concerns and expectations – To begin with you just put down your symptoms to being run down due to work pressures, but as things have got worse you are now worried that there may be something seriously wrong, although you are not sure what this could be. Your American friend's comments have reinforced your concerns. You want the doctor to try to get to the bottom of things.

First words spoken to doctor – 'I've been feeling so tired and run down recently, doctor – I'm worried there's something seriously wrong.'

Medical history – You lost most of your hearing when you were 4 years old and were told this was the result of a severe infection. You have worn hearing aids since then and this has allowed you to maintain your speech, such that you speak almost as clearly as someone without any hearing impairment. You rarely come to see the doctor, other than for smears and minor problems. You have never been depressed.

Drug history – You do not take any regular medication. You do not have any drug allergies.

Social history – You were discouraged from learning sign language when you were a child as your parents were advised that you would be more likely to integrate into a mainstream school if you were forced to lip read. You have never really had any friends within the deaf community. You have never smoked and drink one or two glasses of wine each day over the weekend. You live with Rex, your labrador.

Family history – Your mother had diabetes mellitus, requiring tablets from when she was diagnosed in her 40s. She died aged 62 from a stroke. Your father and brother are fit and well. As far as you know, no one in your family has had heart or cholesterol problems.

- Having read the information given to the simulated patient, what do you now think this station is testing?
- Make notes or discuss your thoughts with a colleague before you turn the page.

Review your approach to this station:

Tested at this station:

1. Diversity issues: communicating with a hearing-impaired patient.
2. History-taking skills.
3. Physical examination.
4. Problem-solving and diagnostic skills.

Domain 1 – Interpersonal skills

Diversity issues: communicating with a hearing-impaired patient

Nine million people in the UK are deaf or hard of hearing. Understanding how to communicate effectively with these patients is a key skill for healthcare professionals:

- The Equality Act (2010), which replaced most of the Disability Discrimination Act 1995, gives equal access to disabled people to services such as healthcare.
- Reasonable adjustments must be made by GPs to allow equitable access to services.
- The GP curriculum points out that reasonable adjustments can be simple strategies such as remembering to always face hard-of-hearing or deaf patients, and to talk slowing and clearly, to allow patients to lip read.
- As you have been made aware of the patient's hearing impairment, you need to be explicit in checking understanding at regular intervals during the consultation. However, it is important to do this in an appropriate and non-patronizing manner.
- An awareness of the needs of hearing-impaired patients and taking simple steps as outlined above can help overcome communication barriers to the doctor–patient relationship.

Domain 2 – Data gathering, technical and assessment skills

History-taking skills

Patients often present with non-specific symptoms such as tiredness. In taking a focused history, you need to tease out relevant symptoms to help reach a working diagnosis:

- She says that she is tired and run down. Can she say more about this?
- How long has she been feeling like this?
- Any other symptoms such as headaches, urinary problems, excessive thirst, bowel disturbance, abdominal pains, weight changes, fevers, cold or heat intolerance, menstrual problems, chest pain, cough or shortness of breath?
- Any visual problems or numbness, pins and needles or weakness in any of her limbs?
- It is always worth asking depression-screening questions to patients who present with non-specific symptoms such as tiredness.

- Has she suffered from any other medical problems in the past?
- Does she take any medication?
- What line of work is she in? Are her symptoms affecting her work?
- Does she smoke? How much alcohol does she drink? Is there anyone at home with her?
- Are there any medical problems in her immediate family, such as diabetes or thyroid problems?
- She says that she is worried that there is something seriously wrong. Does she have any thoughts about what this might be? What does she hope will happen from coming to the surgery today?

Physical examination

From the history you will hopefully have picked up that her symptoms suggest a thyroid disorder. Under the *Metabolic problems* section of the GP curriculum, clinical examination of the neck is listed as a psychomotor skill you should be able to demonstrate. An appropriate focused physical examination at this station should therefore include the neck together with looking for systemic features of thyroid disease:

- Before any physical examination explain to the patient what will be involved and gain verbal consent to proceed.
- Brief systemic thyroid examination could include:
  - Pulse – can be slow and of low volume in hypothyroidism or raised in hyperthyroidism.
  - Is there a tremor? Ask the patient to stretch out their arms in front of them and splay their fingers. Can be present in hyperthyroidism.
  - Loss of the outer third of eyebrows and dry, brittle hair can be present in hypothyroid disease.
  - Eyes – look for exophthalmos (protruding appearance) and lid lag Thyroid eye disease is usually associated with Graves' disease but can occur in chronic autoimmune thyroiditis.
  - Reflexes – may be slow relaxing in hypothyroidism or brisk in hyperthyroidism.
- Examination of the neck:
  - Inspection – any scars? Any thyroid swelling (goitre) visible?
  - If you see a swelling, ask the patient to take a sip of water – a goitre will rise on swallowing.
  - Palpation – best done from behind the patient. Feel for lymph nodes and assess the thyroid gland itself. Is it enlarged? Tender? What is its consistency?
  - Percussion – over the manubrium (upper part of the sternum). If dull this may signify a retrosternal goitre.
  - Auscultation – listening for bruits over the gland.

In the Clinical Skills Assessment (CSA), you will be handed a card if there are any abnormal findings from the examination. *Abnormal findings in this case include a pulse of 48 and a large diffuse goitre.*

Domain 3 – Clinical management skills
Problem-solving and diagnostic skills

The GP curriculum states that thyroid disorders are very common and have an enormous impact on quality of life, but that the diagnosis is often missed. Patients who present with tiredness should always alert you to the possibility of thyroid disease:

- This patient gives a clear history suggesting hypothyroidism.
- Examination findings of bradycardia with a diffuse goitre are also consistent with this diagnosis (see Knowledge base).
- You need to confirm the diagnosis with blood tests – namely, thyroid function tests (TFTs) (see Knowledge base). You should also check glucose, lipid profile, full blood count (FBC) and urea and electrolytes (U&Es).
- You should discuss the probable diagnosis with the patient and explain the need for confirmatory blood tests. Is she happy to have the tests?
- When the patient came into the consultation room she said she was concerned there was something 'seriously wrong'. You need to reassure her that there are no worrying findings and that if an under-active thyroid is confirmed, the condition is common and easily treated with tablets.
- Ask her to return after she has had the blood tests to discuss the results.
- Is she happy with the explanation and plan, and does she have any questions?

Knowledge base - Hypothyroidism

References: NHS Clinical Knowledge Summaries – see Further reading below.

Hypothyroidism	• Under secretion of thyroid hormone • Overt hypothyroidism = thyroid-stimulating hormone (TSH) raised with low free thyroxine (T_4) level • Subclinical hypothyroidism = TSH raised with normal free T_4 level
Causes	• Iodine deficiency (rare in UK) • Autoimmune hypothyroidism (Hashimoto's thyroiditis = autoimmune thyroiditis and goitre) • Post thyroid surgery or radioactive iodine treatment for hyperthyroidism • Drug side effects, e.g. amiodarone and lithium • Secondary to pituitary or hypothalamic disease • Congenital hypothyroidism
How common?	• Approximately 1 in 50 women and 1 in 1000 men develop hypothyroidism during their lifetime
Symptoms and signs	• Generalized tiredness and lethargy, slowing down of mental processes • Cold intolerance • Weight gain • Constipation • Absent, irregular or heavy periods • Dry skin, hair loss and hoarse or deep voice • Carpel tunnel syndrome • Low mood and reduced libido • Diffuse goitre • Myxoedema – non-pitting oedema

(continued)

	• Slowly relaxing tendon reflexes • Bradycardia • Hypercholesterolaemia • Galactorrhoea – secondary to increased prolactin levels
Investigations	• Thyroid function tests: TSH, T_4, free T_4, T_3 and thyroid antibodies
Treatment	• Levothyroxine daily • Start at 50–100 µg OD (25 µg if elderly or ischaemic heart disease) • Monitor TFTs and titrate up every 2–3 months if required
Drug interactions	• Carbamazepine, phenytoin and rifampicin accelerate the metabolism of levothyroxine • Levothyroxine enhances the anticoagulation effects of warfarin • Cimetidine and oral iron reduce absorption of levothyroxine
Free prescriptions	• In England, those receiving levothyroxine are entitled to free prescriptions for all their medicines. (In Scotland, Wales and Northern Ireland prescriptions are free to all.)

Refer patients with hypothyroidism to an endocrinologist if they are under 16 years old, pregnant or postpartum, have ischaemic heart disease, are taking amiodarone or lithium, or if you suspect pituitary or hypothalamic disease.

Take-home messages

- For patients with hearing impairment, making small adjustments within the consultation can significantly improve doctor–patient communication.
- Physical examination skills must be demonstrated by candidates in the CSA.
- The GP curriculum makes clear that management of thyroid disease in primary care is a key competence for general practice.

Tasks

- Re-run the scenario with the patient presenting with symptoms and signs of hyperthyroidism.
- Re-run the scenario with the patient bringing a friend to sign language interpret for her (on the assumption that she can primarily communicate by sign language).
- Re-run the scenario with the patient wearing a hijab (but with no disability). Practise negotiating removal of her hijab for a neck examination.

1-minute explanations for patients

- Explain what hypothyroidism is.
- Explain what hyperthyroidism is.
- Explain the treatment for hyperthyroidism.

Ideas for further revision

Practise mock consultations with a colleague where you imagine that they need to lip read you. Try to modify the consultation and any examination to allow adequate doctor–patient communication.

Further reading

Action on Hearing Loss (formally Royal National Institute for Deaf People) www.actiononhearingloss.org.uk

British Deaf Association (BDA) www.bda.org.uk

British Thyroid Foundation www.btf-thyroid.org

NHS National Library for Health Clinical Knowledge Summaries – hypothyroidism www.cks.library.nhs.uk/hypothyroidism

RCGP curriculum statement 15.6 – Metabolic problems www.rcgp.org.uk

Rehman HU, Bajwa TA. 10-minute consultation: Newly diagnosed hypothyroidism. *BMJ* 2004; 329: 1271 www.bmj.com

Thyroid UK – information and advice for patients www.thyroiduk.org

Information given to candidates

The appointment has been booked by Raymond Mallory's sister, Stephanie Mallory. She wants to talk to you about Raymond, who has Down's syndrome and is a patient at your practice. Raymond's sister lives 70 miles away and is attending on her own today.

Raymond is 44 years old and lives in supported accommodation for people with mild to moderate learning disabilities.

Raymond suffers from diabetes and heart failure, secondary to an incompetent mitral valve. His current medication is:

Spironolactone	25 mg OD	Bisoprolol	10 mg OD
Furosemide	80 mg OD	Metformin	500 mg TDS
Ramipril	5 mg BD	Gliclazide	80 mg OD

The last letter from the cardiologist from a month ago noted that Raymond's heart failure appeared to be gradually deteriorating despite treatment. His renal function is normal and his diabetes well controlled. The cardiologist is due to see him again in 1 month.

Raymond has had three admissions (all less than 1 week's stay) in the last year as a result of worsening breathlessness secondary to heart failure.

On the last admission Raymond was assessed by one of the psychiatrists who judged that he had the capacity to discharge himself early, against medical advice.

Raymond has not appointed anyone to make medical decisions on his behalf (lasting power of attorney).

As Stephanie Mallory enters the room she says, 'Doctor, I want to talk to you about Raymond. He's been so unwell over the last year, the family doesn't think he should go into hospital again if his breathing gets bad.'

- What do you think this station is testing?
- Make notes or discuss your thoughts with a colleague before you read on.

Plan your approach to this station:

Information given to simulated relative

Basic details – You are Stephanie Mallory, a 50-year-old woman and the older sister of Raymond Mallory, who is a patient at the practice. You are attending on your own today. You live 70 miles away and visit Raymond once a month.

Appearance and behaviour – You are well presented and assertive. If the doctor does not agree to your request to keep Raymond out of hospital then you will initially be a little shocked. However, if the doctor explains carefully why this is the case, and takes your perspective and concerns into account, then you will accept this.

History

Freely divulged to doctor – You want to talk to the doctor about your brother, Raymond, who has Down's syndrome. Raymond had an operation on one of his heart valves when he was a baby and over the last 4 years has been suffering from 'heart failure'. He used to see the local heart specialist once every 6 months, as initially things weren't too bad. But now he's very breathless even if he potters around in the garden and his lips always have a bluish tinge. He now sees the heart doctor every 2–3 months.

Divulged to doctor if specifically asked – Raymond is now taking lots of medication, and the heart failure specialist nurse visits every 2–3 weeks to see how he is doing. His ankle swelling seems to have got worse over the last few months, even though Raymond knows that he needs to be careful with how much he drinks. He still seems generally happy and his keyworker – one of the supported accommodation staff – often takes him out on trips or to various groups. Raymond does not seem to know what the heart doctor said to him when he last saw her 1 month ago. Raymond knows that his heart is not working properly and that he has to take all his tablets to help it. You have not discussed with Raymond what he would like to happen if his breathing gets bad again. You have only discussed this with one of Raymond's three brothers. Raymond does not know that you are coming to see the doctor today.

Ideas, concerns and expectations – You still feel a little guilty about moving so far away when your partner got a new job 4 years ago. Raymond has always disliked going into hospital. But over the last year he has become more and more distressed when he has gone in, so much so that the last time he was admitted he came home early, against medical advice. With his worsening condition, and his dislike of hospitals, you believe he should not have to undergo this trauma again if his breathing deteriorates, and should instead be kept at home. You want the doctor to agree with you today that Raymond will stay at home if his breathing gets bad again rather than going into hospital, and you would like this written in his notes.

First words spoken to doctor – 'Doctor, I want to talk to you about Raymond. He's been so unwell over the last year, the family doesn't think he should go into hospital again if his breathing gets bad.'

Medical history – You are fit and well. Raymond suffers from 'heart failure' and diabetes.

Drug history – You do not take any medication. You know that Raymond is on 'lots of tablets' for his heart failure and diabetes.

Social history – You live 70 miles away with your own family. You work as a primary school teacher.

Family history – Apart from Raymond's problems, there are no other significant medical problems in your immediate family.

- Having read the information given to the simulated relative, what do you now think this station is testing?
- Make notes or discuss your thoughts with a colleague before you turn the page.

Review your approach to this station:

Tested at this station:

1. Addressing a relative's concerns.
2. Data gathering.
3. Respecting patient autonomy.
4. Negotiating with a patient's relative.

Domain 1 – Interpersonal skills

Addressing a relative's concerns

This station is primarily about addressing the concerns of a patient's close relative, while respecting patient autonomy and confidentiality in negotiating a way forward. As such, your ability to relate to Raymond's sister in an empathetic and supportive way is a key skill:

- Raymond's sister is obviously concerned about her brother's well-being. You should acknowledge this and ask her to say more about her worries.
- She mentions him being 'so unwell' over the last year. Can she say more about this?
- Is there any particular reason why she is so worried about him going into hospital again? Did anything happen in the last few admissions which upset or concerned her?
- What sort of impact has Raymond's learning disability had on her life?
- Has it been difficult balancing her own life with helping support Raymond?
- Has Raymond ever mentioned what he would like done if his health deteriorates further?
- Has she discussed this matter with anyone else?

Domain 2 – Data gathering, technical and assessment skills

Data gathering

It would be useful to obtain further details about Raymond's health, to help inform you when negotiating a way forward with his sister:

- How is Raymond doing at the moment?
- What is he able to do, what is he not able to do? Is he getting out?
- How have things changed over the last year?
- Does Raymond understand what is happening with his heart problem?
- Is he taking his medication as prescribed?
- Has Raymond said anything that might make you think his poor health is getting him down?
- Has his behaviour changed in any way recently?

Domain 3 – Clinical management skills

Respecting patient autonomy

All adult patients have a right to respect for autonomy (self-determination):

- Under the Mental Capacity Act 2005 for England and Wales, adult patients are presumed to have capacity to make decisions for themselves unless proven otherwise.
- Stephanie Mallory is asking you to make an advance decision regarding withholding care from Raymond, should his condition deteriorate. You are not in a position to agree to this request without consulting Raymond himself.
- Just because a patient has a learning disability does not mean they are incapable of making decisions regarding their medical care. Indeed, Raymond was judged to have the capacity to agree his own discharge during his last admission.
- Although Stephanie believes she has Raymond's best interests at heart, and is a close relative, she has no legal right to determine Raymond's medical treatment.
- Nonetheless, it is good practice to involve relatives in key decisions, with the patient's consent.
- Given Raymond's gradual deterioration, it would be good practice to discuss with him his wishes should he become very ill.

Negotiating with a patient's relative

Although you are not able to agree to Stephanie's request that you keep Raymond at home if he becomes unwell again, you should focus on positive ways forward, emphasizing the need to involve Raymond at all stages:

- You need to sensitively explain that it is important to involve Raymond in any decisions about his future care.
- You could suggest that Stephanie first discusses the issue with Raymond – what would he want to happen if he became ill again? What did he think about being in hospital?
- You could also suggest that Stephanie speaks with Raymond's brothers – what are their thoughts on the matter?
- Involving his keyworker might also be useful – Stephanie could ask her whether Raymond has ever talked about his wishes if he became ill again.
- You could offer to see Raymond to discuss things further. If Raymond is happy, you could see them both together. And you could ask the heart failure nurse specialist to attend, too, if Raymond is ok with this.
- Raymond and his sister may also find it helpful to discuss the issue with his cardiologist at the next appointment.
- You need to be careful to not breach patient confidentiality when negotiating how best to proceed.

Knowledge base

References: see Further reading below

Common and/or important conditions associated with learning disabilities

- *Epilepsy* – increased incidence and complexity with severity of learning disability.
- *Sensory impairments* – hearing and vision, ear wax.
- *Obesity* – predisposes to other medical problems.

- *Gastrointestinal* – swallowing problems, reflux oesophagitis, *Helicobacter pylori* infection, constipation, gastric carcinoma.
- *Respiratory problems* – chest infections, aspiration pneumonia.
- *Cerebral palsy* – especially with severe learning disability.
- *Orthopaedic problems* – joint contractures, osteoporosis.
- *Dermatological problems.*
- *Psychiatric problems* – emotional and behavioural disorders, bereavement reactions, anxiety and depression, schizophrenia, bipolar affective disorder, Alzheimer's disease, autistic spectrum disorder.

Diagnostic overshadowing

The GP curriculum warns against 'diagnostic overshadowing', which is when the presenting complaint of a patient with a learning disability is put down to their learning disability rather than health professionals looking for another cause.

If a patient with a learning disability presents with a new behaviour, or existing ones escalate, you should not dismiss these symptoms as simply due to their learning disability but consider physical, psychiatric and social causes:

- Physical and psychiatric causes – see above.
- Social causes – change in carers, bereavement, abuse.

Take-home messages

- Patients with learning disabilities have the same right to respect for patient autonomy as other patients.
- Make sure you involve patients with learning disabilities as fully as possible in decisions about their care.
- When those close to patients consult you about their relative's/spouse's care, you need to address their concerns in an empathic and supportive way.

Tasks

- Re-run the scenario with Raymond's housing keyworker attending on her own, asking what they should do if Raymond's breathing worsens.
- Re-run the scenario with Raymond and Stephanie attending together to discuss making an advance directive.
- Re-run the scenario with Raymond attending on his own with ear wax. What other issues might you want to discuss?
- For MRCGP[INT] candidates there may be differences in the degree of patient autonomy and the position of relatives in relation to power of attorney and other country-specific legal issues. Re-run the scenario focusing on how the relative feels in relation to the hospital event, discussing what to do if Raymond becomes breathless again and raising the possibility of his death.

1-minute explanations for patients

- Explain what Down's syndrome is.
- Explain what lasting power of attorney is.
- Explain to a relative how capacity is assessed.

Ideas for further revision

Some Clinical Skills Assessment (CSA) stations will primarily be concerned with issues around professionalism and ethics. These topics are specifically covered in the GP curriculum. You should be familiar with the curriculum document and also with key professional guidelines, including those related to confidentiality and consent.

Further reading

e-GP resource has e-learning modules covering the RCGP curriculum, including several on the care of patients with learning disabilities www.e-gp.org

General Medical Council. *Confidentiality.* London: GMC, 2009 www.gmc-uk.org

General Medical Council. *Consent: patients and doctors making decisions together.* London: GMC, 2008 www.gmc-uk.org

Lindsay P (ed). *The Care of the Adult with Intellectual Disability in Primary Care.* Oxford: Radcliffe Press, 2011

RCGP curriculum statement 3.3 – Clinical ethics and values-based practice www.rcgp.org.uk

RCGP curriculum statement 14 – Care of people with learning disabilities www.rcgp.org.uk

STATION 20

Information given to candidates

Margaret Stewart is a 58-year-old female patient who rarely comes to the surgery.

She has been taking enalapril 20 mg for hypertension for 2 years and her blood pressure (BP) is well controlled on medication.

As she enters the consultation room the patient says, 'This ringing in my ears is really getting me down, doctor.'

- What do you think this station is testing?
- Make notes or discuss your thoughts with a colleague before you read on.

Plan your approach to this station:

Information given to simulated patient

Basic details – You are Margaret Stewart, a divorced 58-year-old social worker.

Appearance and behaviour – You are articulate and well presented, with good eye contact throughout the consultation.

History

Freely divulged to doctor – You noticed a ringing sound in both ears about 3 months ago. It came on gradually over a few weeks. It has not really changed since then. It is not something you have ever had before and it is now interfering with your life and making you frustrated. You have not mentioned this to anyone else. You put off coming down to the surgery as you 'don't like to bother' the doctor and thought that it would probably just go away on its own.

Divulged to doctor if specifically asked – The ringing noise worries you, and the more you worry, the more you focus on the noise. Your house is quiet at night and this is when you feel the ringing is loudest. Your sleep has been disturbed over the last 2 months as you find yourself thinking about the ringing when you are trying to get off to sleep. You consider yourself 'a bit of a worrier'. You did not want to trouble other people, so you have not discussed this with your daughter or friends. You have never had your ears syringed for wax and cannot remember the last time you even had an ear infection. Your hearing does not seem to be any worse than normal. You are eating well, you get pleasure from seeing your family, and enjoy dealing with clients at work, although the management side is quite stressful. You have not had any ear pain or discharge. You have not noticed any weakness in your facial muscles, or any other symptoms in the rest of your body. You have not felt dizzy or noticed a problem with your balance. Although you have got frustrated with the ringing, you do not think you are depressed. You have not banged your head recently and have not been suffering from a cold.

Ideas, concerns and expectations – You were very close to your grandfather when you were younger. You remember that he always complained about his ears. You were 8 years old when your mother told you that he had died from a brain tumour, and since the problem with your ears started you have been worried that the same thing might be happening to you. You are keen for the doctor to explain to you what is going on and ideally reassure you that it is not anything serious. You will be happy to try any self-help measures that the doctor suggests.

First words spoken to doctor – 'This ringing in my ears is really getting me down, doctor.'

Medical history – Two years ago you were found to have high BP. You spent a few months trying to bring the BP down by adopting a healthier lifestyle, but this did not seem to work so you started taking tablets. The medication appears to have worked as the nurse always says things are fine at your 6-monthly check-ups. Apart from minor illnesses you have otherwise been fit and well. You have never suffered from depression.

Drug history – You take BP medication – enalapril 20 mg once a day – for high BP. You are not allergic to any medication.

Social history – You are a full-time social worker. The job has been getting more and more stressful over recent years, particularly since you were promoted to team leader 3 years ago. You split up with your husband 10 years ago and now live on your own. You have one adult daughter who lives nearby and has her own family – a partner and two boys. You have never smoked. You drink less than a bottle of wine a week.

Family history – There are no major health problems in your immediate family.

- Having read the information given to the simulated patient, what do you now think this station is testing?
- Make notes or discuss your thoughts with a colleague before you turn the page.

Review your approach to this station:

Tested at this station:

1. Identifying a hidden agenda.
2. History-taking skills.
3. Physical examination.
4. Management of common medical conditions presenting in primary care.

Domain I – Interpersonal skills

Identifying a hidden agenda

This patient is concerned that she has a brain tumour. However, you are unlikely to uncover this unless you elicit her thoughts about what happened to her grandfather:

- In the Clinical Skills Assessment be alert to cues – either verbal or non-verbal – from the patient.
- Just a simple 'Have you any concerns?' may not be enough to elicit a patient's deepest fears.
- Use good listening skills, go at the patient's pace and be empathic. The patient will be more likely to open up if you adopt such an approach.
- When you are trying to identify a patient's ideas, concerns and expectations, it is often useful to ask whether any friends or family members have experienced similar symptoms. What happened to them? Does the patient think the same might happen to her?
- If you are half-way through a CSA station but get the sense that you are missing some key element to the consultation, it is worth revisiting the patient's ideas, concerns and expectations. At this stage, questions such as *'Is there anything else you would like to tell me?'* can prove fruitful.

Domain 2 – Data gathering, technical and assessment skills

History-taking skills

Although the causes of tinnitus are usually benign, it is important to take a thorough history to try to exclude serious causes (see Knowledge base below) and to assess the impact on the patient's life:

- Start with open questions. Can she say more about the ringing in her ears? In what way is it getting her down? How is she coping with the noise? What are her thoughts about what is going on? What was she hoping would happen from coming to the surgery today?
- More specific questions that you could ask include:
  - Is the ringing in both ears or just one?
  - Is it present all the time, or does it come and go?
  - How long has she noticed the ringing?
  - What makes it better, what makes it worse?
  - Any associated symptoms with the ringing?

- How intrusive does she find the noise? Does it affect her sleep?
- Does it stop her doing things?
- Any previous ear problems? How is her hearing?
- What medication has she taken over the last 6 months?
- Any previous exposure to high levels of noise? What is her job?
- How are things at home?
- Any major life events recently?
- Has she banged her head recently?

Physical examination

At this station you would be expected to examine the patient's ears and test her hearing – see station 6. You should also examine her cranial nerves, particularly V and VII (see Further reading).

You will be told that all the examinations are normal.

Domain 3 – Clinical management skills

Management of common medical conditions presenting in primary care

The patient is experiencing bilateral tinnitus (the perception of noise with no external stimulus):

- You should reassure her that although the noise can be distressing, it is common and there are a number of ways to help with the condition.
- Explicitly address her fear about it being cancer and explain that none of the symptoms or signs suggests anything serious.
- You could suggest organizing some simple blood tests – full blood count (FBC), thyroid function tests (TFTs) and random glucose – to ensure that you are not missing any general health problem. What does the patient think about this?
- You could offer to refer her for a formal hearing test (audiometry), however in this case the patient reports that her hearing has not got worse.
- The GP curriculum states that with tinnitus you should try to empower patients to adopt self-treatment and coping strategies, where appropriate. Self-help advice which you could discuss with the patient includes:
  - general sleep hygiene measures, e.g. avoiding caffeine in the evening, trying to do some exercise during the day and winding down before bedtime
  - background noise – this will help focus the brain away from the tinnitus (e.g. radio hiss, leaving windows open, using a fan)
  - joining a local self-help group for further advice and support, such as those run by the British Tinnitus Association (see Further reading below).
- Ask to see the patient again for a review in a month's time, or sooner if she has any concerns or new symptoms. Explain that if the tinnitus continues to cause problems despite self-help measures, there is the option of referral for tinnitus retraining therapy, which includes cognitive behaviour therapy and sound therapy (e.g. white noise generators or hearing aids to increase background noise).
- Referral to an ear, nose and throat (ENT) specialist would also be an option if the ringing continues to be intrusive.

Knowledge base – Tinnitus

References: NHS Clinical Knowledge Summaries, *BMJ* tinnitus article – see Further reading below.

	Associated with tinnitus
More commonly	• Presbyacusis – age-related hearing loss • Long-term exposure to excessive noise, e.g. occupational hazard, non-use of ear protectors • Middle-ear infections • Perforated tympanic membrane • Meniere's disease • Damage to the cochlear or other inner-ear apparatus • Otosclerosis • Anaemia • Excessive wax
Less commonly	• Exposure to sudden or very loud noise, e.g. gunfire, explosion • Head injury • Impacted wisdom teeth • Medication, e.g. loop diuretics, tricyclics, quinine, aminoglycosides, aspirin, non-steroidal anti-inflammatory drugs (NSAIDs) • Solvent or alcohol misuse • High blood pressure • Hyperthyroidism
Rarely	• Acoustic neuroma

Refer to a specialist if:
● objective tinnitus (can be heard by an observer)
● pulsatile tinnitus (unless due to an acute inflammatory ear infection)
● unilateral tinnitus without an obvious cause (such as exposure to a recent loud noise on that side)
● persistent intrusive tinnitus
● associated deafness.

Take-home messages
• If you are patient-centred during consultations then the patient's agenda is more likely to be revealed.
• You need to feel confident in the management of common conditions presenting in primary care.
• Always remember to 'safety-net' with appropriate follow-up or explicit instructions on when patients should re-present.

Tasks
● Re-run the scenario with the patient presenting with unilateral tinnitus. How might this affect your data gathering and management?

- Re-run the scenario with the patient having a perforation of her right pars flaccida. How might this change the management options?
- Re-run the scenario with the patient demanding a referral to a specialist.
- A particular difficulty is eliciting concerns. As we point out, asking 'Have you any concerns?' may not be enough to uncover a patient's deepest fears. Practise role-playing alternative ways of identifying concerns, e.g. picking up and reflecting back any verbal cues, or commenting on signs of anxiety in her body language.

1-minute explanations for patients

- Explain what tinnitus is.
- Explain why it's not usual practice to refer all patients with tinnitus to an ENT specialist.
- Explain how background noise (e.g. radio hiss) may help.

Ideas for further revision

The CSA uses a series of blueprints to ensure that for each 13-station examination there is a range of complexity in the cases. There will also be a balance to the nature of cases (e.g. acute problems, chronic disease management, diversity and ethical issues, etc.). Furthermore, each CSA will contain stations covering a variety of systems (e.g. ENT, cardiovascular, respiratory, women's health, etc.). Try to ensure your revision takes account of all these dimensions, and use the GP curriculum to identify gaps in your knowledge.

Further reading

British Tinnitus Association – information sheets for patients and health professionals www.tinnitus.org.uk

ENT UK – includes patient information on a range of ENT conditions www.entuk.org

Hannan SA, Sami F, Wareing MJ. 10-minute consultation – tinnitus. *BMJ* 2005: 330; 237 www.bmj.com

NHS National Library for Health Clinical Knowledge Summaries – Tinnitus www.cks.nhs.uk/tinnitus

RCGP curriculum statement 15.4 – Clinical management: ENT and facial problems www.rcgp.org.uk

Thomas J, Monaghan T. *Oxford Handbook of Clinical Examination and Practical Skills*. Oxford: Oxford University Press, 2007

Information given to candidates

Angus Henderson is a 32-year-old patient who has been registered with the practice for 8 years but has attended on only three occasions – once for a life insurance medical check and twice for minor, self-limiting illnesses.

As the patient enters the room he says, 'I'm sorry to waste your time, doctor, but my wife made me come down. Things have been a bit blurry in my right eye – just the central bit – for a few weeks, but it's back to normal now and I'm sure it's nothing to worry about. I just need to get my eyes checked at the optician, don't you think?'

- What do you think this station is testing?
- Make notes or discuss your thoughts with a colleague before you read on.

Plan your approach to this station:

Information given to simulated patient

Basic details – You are Angus Henderson, a 32-year-old bus driver.

Appearance and behaviour – You come across as being dismissive that there might be anything seriously wrong. Deep down you are in fact worried, but you are overcompensating for this by your unconcerned, nonchalant attitude with the doctor today. You will try to cajole the doctor into agreeing with you that all is well. If the doctor is caring and empathetic, but clear in explaining that your symptoms cannot be so easily dismissed, you will be inclined to disclose your true concerns and ask the doctor directly if you could have multiple sclerosis.

History

Freely divulged to doctor – Four weeks ago you noticed a problem with the vision in your right eye. If you covered up your left eye there seemed to be a central patch that was very blurred. Your left eye was fine and things cleared up completely within 3 weeks. You have had floaters in both eyes in the past and so dismissed it as probably being due to a large floater, although you have never had a floater that big and previously floaters have not made your vision blurred. Your vision is back to normal now.

Divulged to doctor if specifically asked – Your right eye was painful if you moved it during the time when your vision was affected. You nearly had an accident while driving your bus at work a couple of weeks ago when the car in front braked suddenly just as you were scratching your left eyelid. You did not see the car properly until you opened your left eye, due to the blurred vision. You have not had headaches or any weakness in your limbs or face. If the doctor specifically asks about times in the past when you may have had sensory symptoms, you will remember that a couple of years ago you had tingling sensations and some numbness in the toes of your left foot for about a week, which you put down to a new pair of tight shoes. You have had no such symptoms since. Your speech has been normal. You have not had any bladder or bowel problems.

Ideas, concerns and expectations – You think of yourself as extremely fit and healthy – it has been years since you came to see the doctor and you have never been in hospital. Deep down you are concerned that you are suffering from something serious – you had heard about multiple sclerosis on the radio and know that it can start with eye problems. You have been coping with these fears by convincing yourself that there is nothing really to worry about as things have resolved completely and you are in such good health generally. You have not discussed your fears with your wife, but she made you book an appointment at the surgery as she knew about the blurred vision and insisted you should get things checked out. You want the doctor to go along with your expressed view that this is nothing serious, as this will allay your fears. To this end you will underplay the visual problem you have had, unless the doctor asks specific questions about your symptoms.

First words spoken to doctor – 'I'm sorry to waste your time, doctor, but my wife made me come down. Things have been a bit blurry in my right eye – just the central bit – for a few weeks, but it's back to normal now and I'm sure it's nothing to worry about. I just need to get my eyes checked at the optician, don't you think?'

Medical history – Apart from the tingling sensation and numbness in your toes a couple of years ago, you are fit and well. You have been to the doctor's only three times in the last 8 years – once for a life insurance medical and twice for coughs and colds.

Drug history – You do not take any regular medication and you have no drug allergies.

Social history – You are married with three young children. You go running three or four times a week. You drink the odd pint of beer at the weekend, unless you are working. You have never smoked.

Family history – There is no history of any of your family having eye or major health problems.

- Having read the information given to the simulated patient, what do you now think this station is testing?
- Make notes or discuss your thoughts with a colleague before you turn the page.

Review your approach to this station:

Tested at this station:

1. Dealing with a dismissive patient.
2. History-taking skills.
3. Physical examination.
4. Reaching a shared management plan.

Domain 1 – Interpersonal skills

Dealing with a dismissive patient

This patient has significant recent symptoms that he is trying to trivialize in an attempt to allay his fears that there may be something seriously wrong:

- This patient wants you to agree with him that the recent episode of blurred vision is nothing to worry about. He will try to play down the extent and severity of his symptoms and encourage you to confirm that a visit to the optician is all that is required.
- In one sense he is superficially in denial about his symptoms. Denial can be a powerful coping mechanism when patients are confronted with the potentially serious implications of certain symptoms or diagnoses. However, on another level he is aware and frightened at the implications of his blurred vision, although he has tried to suppress these concerns, even to himself.
- Initially the patient will be quite manipulative in trying to get you to agree that this is only a minor problem and that all is well. In response, you need to be clear that you do not think this is something that can so readily be dismissed.
- The key here is to be able to feel comfortable in disagreeing with the patient, albeit in a professional and non-confrontational manner. Responses such as *'Well, I'm not so sure'* or *'I can see why you might believe that but I don't think we can just dismiss your symptoms without further investigations'* may be useful.
- You will have to employ all your interpersonal skills to try to tease out his true concerns. You need to demonstrate to him through active listening, non-verbal communication and a caring, empathic approach that you are a doctor he can open up to.
- Probing his thoughts about what has happened may also help. Why does he think the blurred vision is a minor problem? Did he ever think this might be something more serious? What does he think caused the symptoms?

Domain 2 – Data gathering, technical and assessment skills

History-taking skills

The patient has presented with a worrying neurological symptom, albeit one that appears to have resolved. This case tests your ability to take a detailed history to try to uncover whether the patient has experienced any other neurological deficits in the past, to help narrow down the differential diagnoses:

- He mentions having some blurred vision in his right eye. Can he say more about this?
- When did he first notice this? What was it like?
- Did he have any other eye symptoms, such as pain or double vision?

- Was his eye red and inflamed?
- What has his left eye been like?
- How and when did his symptoms resolve?
- Has anything like this ever happened before?
- Does he suffer from headaches?
- Any weakness, numbness or odd sensations in his face or any of his limbs? Looking back, can he think of any episodes when he may have had funny sensations, numbness or weakness?
- Has he been affected by problems with his balance or dizziness recently or in the past?
- Any difficulty with swallowing or speech? Any memory problems?
- Any bowel, bladder or erectile problems?
- Were his symptoms worse when it was hot or if he had been exercising?
- Has he had any previous medical problems? Any regular medication?
- Does he smoke? How much alcohol does he drink?
- How has his general health been? Any fatigue or low mood?
- What job does he do?
- How did his blurred vision affect his life – at home and at work?

Physical examination

This is a fairly full station, with candidates having to deal with the patient's dismissive attitude, take a detailed history and address fitness-to-drive issues, all in 10 minutes. Given his presenting complaint, you should say that you would like to perform a full neurological examination and check his blood pressure (BP). However, you will not be required to actually perform the examinations but will be told: *There is pallor of the right optic disc on fundoscopy. All other findings on examination of the cranial and peripheral nervous system including visual acuity and visual fields are normal. BP today is 128/82 mmHg.*

Domain 3 – Clinical management skills

Reaching a shared management plan

Initially there may be discordance between the patient's dismissive attitude and your concerns. But if you have managed to uncover his deep-seated worries, you will be in a better position to negotiate a management plan acceptable to both of you:

- His recent visual symptoms and examination findings are consistent with a diagnosis of optic neuritis, which is associated with multiple sclerosis.
- He experienced an episode of tingling sensations and numbness in the toes of his left foot a couple of years ago, although this could have been due to his footwear.
- Even though you may suspect a serious neurological condition, such as multiple sclerosis, from the history, it would be premature to mention a specific diagnosis to the patient at this stage. Doing so would have significant implications for the patient and you should wait for specialist input and further assessment.
- However, if he asks you directly if it could be multiple sclerosis then you would have to reply honestly and say that it is one possibility, although you should share your uncertainty with him at this stage.
- Although multiple sclerosis is still a clinical diagnosis based on two episodes involving at least two parts of the central nervous system separated in time, the

McDonald criteria (see Further reading) allow earlier diagnosis, in some cases, by incorporating imaging and laboratory tests. This has the potential to facilitate earlier decisions on treatment options.

- Hence if you suspect multiple sclerosis, you should be looking to refer to a neurologist without delay.
- How does the patient feel about being referred to see a specialist?
- Does he understand that it is currently unclear what caused his visual problems but that it is important to look into this further? What are his thoughts about this?
- In the meantime you could suggest some simple screening blood tests, e.g. full blood count (FBC), thyroid function tests (TFTs), glucose, vitamin B12 and folate. Is he ok with having these?
- You could advise the patient that the specialist might decide to organize – a magnetic resonance imaging (MRI) scan – and describe what that would be like for the patient, e.g. *'like going into a long doughnut which makes funny noises, for about 15 minutes'*. Explain that the specialist may also want to take a sample of fluid from his spine together with further eye tests.
- There are Driver and Vehicle Licensing Agency (DVLA) issues. Although the patient's visual deficit seems to have resolved, this has only been grossly tested by you today and needs further assessment. The patient has recently nearly had an accident and given that he drives a bus and is responsible for the safety of his passengers, you should advise him to refrain from driving until he sees the neurologist. If a diagnosis of multiple sclerosis is subsequently made then he would need to inform the DVLA, which would then decide whether he is medically fit to drive.
- Refraining from driving has major implications for this patient and you should explore his thoughts and feelings about this measure.

Knowledge base

Reference: DVLA guidance – see Further reading below.

		Group 1 – includes cars and motor cycles	Group 2 – includes buses and large lorries
Neurological	Epilepsy	6 months off driving after first seizure, unless clinical factors or investigation results which suggest an unacceptably high risk of a further seizure (i.e. ≥20% risk per annum).	Minimum 5 years off driving after first seizure.
	Transient ischaemic attach (TIA) and stroke	Must not drive for at least 1 month. If recovery is satisfactory after a month, then can resume driving.	Licence revoked for at least 1 year. Can be considered for review thereafter if full and complete recovery.
	Multiple sclerosis	Providing medical assessment confirms that driving performance is not impaired, can be licensed. 1-, 2- or 3 licence may be required.	Licence revoked if condition is progressive or disabling.

(continued)

		Group 1 – includes cars and motor cycles	Group 2 – includes buses and large lorries
Vision	Acuity	Must be able to read a number plate at a distance of 20 m.	New applicants are barred if corrected visual acuity is worse than 6/9 in the better eye or 6/12 in the other eye. The uncorrected acuity in each eye must be at least 3/60.
Cardiovascular system	Angina	Stop driving if symptoms occur at rest, with emotion or at the wheel.	Licence revoked if continuing symptoms (treated and/or untreated).
	Acute coronary syndromes	Stop driving for at least 1 week if successfully treated by angioplasty; 4 weeks if not successfully treated by angioplasty. See full guidance for details.	Stop driving for at least 6 weeks.
	Hypertension	Driving may continue unless treatment causes unacceptable side effects.	Disqualified from driving if resting BP consistently ≥180/100 mmHg (either figure).
	Arrhythmias	Stop driving if the arrhythmia has caused, or is likely to cause, incapacity.	Disqualified from driving if the arrhythmia has caused or is likely to cause incapacity.
Diabetes mellitus	Diet or tablet controlled	No restrictions unless develop sequelae, e.g. diabetic eye disease affecting vision, or have more than one episode of hypoglycaemia requiring the assistance of another person within the preceding 12 months.	Various criteria must be met, including: no episode of hypoglycaemia requiring the assistance of another person has occurred in the preceding 12 months; regular monitoring of blood glucose; full awareness of hypoglycaemia. See full guidance for details.
	Controlled by insulin	Various criteria must be met, including: must have awareness of hypoglycaemia; must not have had more than one episode of hypoglycaemia requiring the assistance of another person in the preceding 12 months; there must be appropriate blood glucose monitoring; must not be regarded as a likely source of danger to the public while driving; the visual standards for acuity and visual field must be met. See full guidance for details.	From 15 November 2011, may apply for any Group 2 licence. However, must satisfy the criteria listed in the box above, plus additional requirements. See full guidance for details.

(continued)

(continued)

		Group 1 – includes cars and motor cycles	Group 2 – includes buses and large lorries
Psychiatric disorders	Acute psychotic disorder	Driving must cease during the acute illness. Re-licensing can be considered when well for at least 3 months, compliant with treatment, free from adverse effects of medication which would impair driving and subject to a favourable specialist report.	Driving must cease pending a medical enquiry. Normally required to be well and stable for 3 years before driving can be resumed.
	Dementia	Very difficult to assess. In early dementia when sufficient skills are retained and progression is slow, a licence may be issued subject to annual review.	Licence revoked.
Respiratory and sleep disorders	Chronic obstructive pulmonary disease (COPD) and asthma	DVLA need not be notified unless attacks are associated with disabling giddiness, fainting or loss of consciousness.	As for Group 1.
	Obstructive sleep apnoea	Stop driving until satisfactory control of symptoms attained.	Stop driving until satisfactory control of symptoms and ongoing compliance with treatment, confirmed by specialist.

Take-home messages

- Patients who appear dismissive about potentially serious symptoms may be using denial as a coping mechanism.
- Explore their health beliefs thoroughly but make clear that you do not agree that their symptoms can be so readily dismissed.
- You have a responsibility to advise patients to refrain from driving and contact the DVLA if you believe that their medical condition places them or others at risk.

Tasks

- Re-run the scenario with the patient complaining of ongoing blurred vision in his right eye. How might this affect management options?
- Re-run the scenario with the patient telling you that he will let the DVLA know but feels that he can't let his colleagues down, so he plans to finish his last three shifts at work this week.
- Re-run the scenario with the patient presenting with a short history of tingling and numbness of his right arm only.

1-minute explanations for patients

- Explain what happens when you have an MRI scan.
- Explain how the DVLA determines someone's fitness to drive.
- Explain what might be the differential diagnoses in this case.

Ideas for further revision

The GP curriculum states that one of the psychomotor skills you must be able to demonstrate is competence in performing a full neurological examination. Although not required at this station, this can be readily tested in the Clinical Skills Assessment (CSA), so practise with colleagues until you feel confident in your ability to perform a slick neurological examination.

Further reading

DVLA Swansea. *For Medical Practitioners: At a glance guide to the current medical standards of fitness to drive.* August 2011 www.dft.gov.uk/dvla/medical/ataglance.aspx

General Medical Council. Supplementary Guidance: Confidentiality – reporting concerns about patients to the DVLA or the DVA. London, 2009 www.gmc-uk.org

Multiple Sclerosis Society UK – information for patients and professionals www.mssociety.org.uk

Nicholas R, Chataway J. Multiple sclerosis. Clinical evidence. BMJ Evidence Centre, May 2009 clinicalevidence.bmj.com/ceweb/conditions/nud/1202/1202.jsp

Polman C, *et al.* Diagnostic criteria for multiple sclerosis: 2010 revisions to the McDonald criteria. *Annals of Neurology*, 2011; 69: 292–302

Information given to candidates

Candidates note: this station is an out-of-hours **home visit**. You will be escorted by one of the invigilators to a room made to look like a patient's sitting room. The consultation will take place there.

You are working a Saturday morning session for the local out-of-hours provider.

Your first call of the day is a home visit to see Ben Wayne, a 74-year-old patient at a neighbouring practice to your own.

You do not have access to his GP medical records.

The information provided by the out-of-hours triage service states:

Patient	Ben Wayne
Age	74 years old
Problem	Patient describes chest pain at approximately 2 am last night. Not sure how long it lasted. Patient thought it was indigestion. Did not radiate to arms or neck. No shortness of breath. Patient says he feels fine now.
History	No history of heart problems. Has had 'camera test of stomach' due to indigestion last year.
Medication	Lansoprazole 15 mg OD
Management	Patient advised to call 999 and go straight to hospital for investigation and treatment. Patient refused admission, stating he is now well and just wants 'checking over'. Agreed to home visit.

The first words from the patient as you enter the room are, 'I'm sorry about all the fuss, doctor, I know they wanted me to go to hospital but I'm feeling fine now and there's no way I'm going to miss seeing my new granddaughter.'

- What do you think this station is testing?
- Make notes or discuss your thoughts with a colleague before you read on.

Plan your approach to this station:

Information given to simulated patient

Basic details – You are Ben Wayne, a 74-year-old retired plumber.

Appearance and behaviour – You are a little flustered at the events of last night together with your planned trip by train to see your new granddaughter.

History

Freely divulged to doctor – You woke up at 2 am earlier today with chest pain. The pain was constant and lasted about 45 minutes. Initially you thought it was indigestion, but it did not go away or change when you sat up or moved around. You had a glass of water and some paracetamol, but nothing seemed to make any difference to the pain. You started to get worried when the pain was still there after half an hour. By then you thought that it might be a heart problem, but now you think it was probably due to stress.

Divulged to doctor if specifically asked – The chest pain felt like severe heavy pressure over the middle of your chest. You felt nauseous and short of breath with the pain. The pain did not radiate to your neck or arms, or go through to your back. You have never experienced a pain like this before. The pain was not worse as you breathed. You have not had any pain in your calves or any leg swelling. You do not have a cough. You felt fit and well until last night. You did not experience any heart palpitations (feeling your heart beating in your chest or a rapid heart beat). The pain gradually started to ease after about 40 minutes and had gone within a further 5 minutes. You were able to go back to sleep after another half an hour. You woke up feeling a little tired, but otherwise ok. There has been no recurrence of the pain. You do not want your daughter to know what has happened.

Ideas, concerns and expectations – You have not told your daughter what happened as you know she will tell you not to travel and you really want to see your first grandchild. You think the pain was probably due to stress over all the travel arrangements. At one point you did think the pain might be coming from your heart, but because it went away and you now feel absolutely fine, you do not think it could be anything serious like a heart attack. But you thought you should speak to someone about it, so you rang your GP surgery in the morning and were transferred through to the out-of-hours service. When they said you should dial 999 and go straight to hospital you thought they were being over-cautious. You told them you did not think you needed to go to hospital, but agreed to a home visit from the doctor. The idea of going to hospital is also distressing as it reminds you of when your wife was very ill. You expect that once the doctor sees how well you are, they won't say that you should go straight to hospital. If the doctor does ask you to go now, you will strongly resist this request. Even if the doctor says you may well have had a heart attack and could risk your life without immediate treatment, you will simply refuse to miss your planned trip. However, if you feel confident in the doctor's abilities then – after some discussion – you will offer to go to see your own GP on your return on Monday morning, and immediately seek help if you have any further episodes of chest pain over the weekend. You will be happy to take any medication that the doctor wants to give you now.

First words spoken to doctor – The first words from the patient as you enter the room are, 'I'm sorry about all the fuss, doctor, I know they wanted me to go to hospital but I'm feeling fine now and there's no way I'm going to miss seeing my new granddaughter.'

Medical history – As far as you know, you have never had high blood pressure or any heart problems. You suffered from quite severe indigestion last year, but after having a 'camera test' and taking some tablets to get rid of 'a bug in my stomach', you have been much better. You do not recall having had your cholesterol checked.

Drug history – You take one tablet every morning for indigestion – lansoprazole 15 mg. You have no allergies.

Social history – You live on your own. Your wife died 10 years ago from breast cancer and you are very close to your only daughter who moved last year and now lives 60 miles away. You worked as a plumber until retirement 10 years ago. You gave up smoking 2 years ago but had been a heavy smoker for 30 years (about 40 cigarettes a day). You want to cut down on fried foods and eat a healthier diet.

Family history – Your father died from a stroke aged 62 and your older brother had a heart attack aged 53.

- Having read the information given to the simulated patient, what do you now think this station is testing?
- Make notes or discuss your thoughts with a colleague before you turn the page.

Review your approach to this station:

Tested at this station:

1. Understanding the patient's perspective and respecting patient autonomy.
2. History-taking skills.
3. Physical examination.
4. Recognition and management of a potentially life-threatening condition.
5. Negotiating a management plan.

Domain 1 – Interpersonal skills

Understanding the patient's perspective and respecting patient autonomy

Competent, fully informed patients have a right to refuse treatment, even if this puts them at risk of serious harm. Eliciting the patient's ideas, concerns and expectations will help you understand his perspective on events:

- The GP curriculum states that GPs should be able to deal sensitively and in line with professional codes of practice with patients who may have a serious diagnosis and refuse admission.
- You need to try to find out why the patient is so reluctant to go into hospital. Is it just about missing his trip to see his granddaughter or are there any other concerns? In this case, he has distressing memories associated with hospital visits when his wife was ill.
- This scenario is designed to see whether you can respect patient autonomy where a competent patient refuses to comply with your request for his immediate admission to hospital.
- There is a tension between your judgement of what is in his best interests and his strongly held preference to travel to see his new granddaughter, whatever the risks.
- Although you should be frank with the patient about the potential consequences of going against medical advice, you need to be careful not to be coercive or bullying in your approach.

Domain 2 – Data gathering, technical and assessment skills

History-taking skills

You may feel that from the information given by the out-of-hours triage service, this patient is unlikely to have a serious condition. However, be wary of second-hand histories – these can often change dramatically when you hear the first-hand account (as in this case):

- Any complaint of chest pain needs a thorough history to try to identify life-threatening conditions such as myocardial infarction (MI), pulmonary embolus or dissecting aortic aneurysm.
- In an out-of-hours setting, without access to the patient's medical records, taking a careful history becomes even more important.

- You need to ask various questions about the pain itself (see Knowledge base) as part of a comprehensive cardiovascular history, including risk factors for ischaemic heart disease.

Physical examination

Owing to time constraints at this station, you will not have to examine the patient. However, you would be expected to attempt to examine him, at which point the examiner will tell you the findings – namely, that cardiovascular examination is normal.

Domain 3 – Clinical management skills

Recognition and management of a potentially life-threatening condition

The GP curriculum states that GPs should be competent in the recognition and immediate management of emergencies encountered in primary care (see Knowledge base):

- The history of what happened in the night should alert you to the strong possibility that the patient has had an MI.
- In addition, this patient has a number of risk factors for heart disease, including a family history of cardiovascular disease, 60 pack years accumulated as a smoker and a high-saturated-fat diet.
- You need to make it clear to the examiner that you consider this a potentially life-threatening situation requiring immediate action (see Knowledge base).
- In this case, the management is complicated by the patient's refusal to be admitted to hospital.
- You need to treat him – as far as he will permit – to minimize the risk of cardiac damage.

Negotiating a management plan (overlap with domain 1)

It is essential that you elicit the patient's ideas, concerns and expectations, to allow you to engage with him in a meaningful way and negotiate how to proceed:

- You must not collude with the patient in downplaying the potential seriousness of the current situation.
- You need to be very clear about the fact that he may well have had a heart attack and that he needs immediate assessment in hospital.
- If he is adamant that he does not want to go to hospital, you need to ensure that he understands that this is a potentially life-threatening situation.
- Even though he feels well now, you can explain that he is at very high risk of a further episode, and without appropriate treatment this might prove fatal.
- Would he allow you to contact his daughter, or another member of the family, to discuss what has happened?
- If he continues to refuse to go straight to hospital, even though he is aware of the risks, would he be prepared to go to his daughter's local hospital, once he has seen his granddaughter? Or agree to see his own GP as soon as he returns?
- If he has any further chest pain, your advice must be to seek immediate medical help. Will he agree to this?

- Would he allow you to give him some aspirin now and a spray to use under his tongue if he has any further chest pain? You need to explain why these are important.

Knowledge base

References: include RCGP curriculum statement 7, appendix 3; National Institute for Clinical Excellence (NICE) CG95 – see Further reading below.

'Dangerous' diagnoses	• Certain conditions encountered in primary care require urgent action, including: • Acute coronary syndrome, i.e. MI or unstable angina • pulmonary embolus • carbon monoxide poisoning • subarachnoid haemorrhage • appendicitis • limb ischaemia • intestinal obstruction or perforation • meningococcal and other bacterial septicaemia • aneurysms • ectopic pregnancy • acute psychosis/mania • visual problems that could threaten blindness: • retinal detachment and haemorrhage • temporal arteritis
Cautious approach	• If you suspect any of the diagnoses above, in a primary care setting, you should arrange for the patient to be transferred to a secondary care centre, to allow a more thorough assessment. • At times, you may be seen to be over-cautious, but without the ability to conduct a range of investigations and close monitoring it can be difficult to exclude such life-threatening conditions in primary care.
Immediate management of suspected ACS	• Do not routinely administer oxygen, but if available, offer if: • Spot oxygen concentration (SpO_2) <94% and not at risk of hypercapnic respiratory failure (aim for SpO_2 of 94–98%) • Chronic obstructive pulmonary disease (COPD) and risk of hypercapnic respiratory failure (aim for SpO_2 of 88–92%) • Give aspirin 300 mg • Pain relief: GTN and/or an intravenous opioid • A resting 12-lead electrocardiogram (ECG) (but do not delay transfer to hospital to perform)
Pain history	• A useful mnemonic when obtaining a detailed history of chest – and other – pain is: **SSS, OPD, RAAT** • Site – where exactly is the pain? • Sort – what does the pain feel like – sharp, dull, tight, etc.? • Severity – on a scale of 1 to 10, how bad is the pain? • Onset – when did the pain start and what was the patient doing? • Periodicity – does the pain come and go or is it constant? • Duration – how long does the pain last? • Radiation – does the pain radiate anywhere? • Alleviating or worsening factors – what makes the pain better? What makes it worse? • Associated symptoms – e.g. nausea, sweating, breathlessness • Time off work – how has the pain affected the patient's life?

> **Take-home messages**
> - You need to take a detailed history for all complaints of chest pain.
> - Patient autonomy must be respected in competent, fully informed patients.
> - You should feel confident in the initial management of life-threatening conditions seen in primary care.

Tasks

- Re-run the scenario with the patient's chest pain occurring >72 hours ago (see NICE guidance).
- Re-run the scenario with the patient collapsing as you take the history. For example, a manikin may appear – do you know the current Basic Life Support guidance? Can you demonstrate it?
- Re-run the scenario as a telephone consultation. Think what other options you might present to the patient if he continues to refuse to go to hospital.
- Re-run the scenario with the patient attending your practice with chest pain but refusing to go to hospital.

1-minute explanations for patients

- Explain what a heart attack is.
- Explain why you need to give aspirin.
- Explain how a GTN spray works.

Ideas for further revision

Learning objectives in the GP curriculum, which the Clinical Skills Assessment (CSA) will base scenarios around, include the immediate management of acutely ill people. In this context, the curriculum states that specific psychomotor skills you should be able to demonstrate include:

- cardiopulmonary resuscitation of children and adults including use of a defibrillator
- performing and interpreting an ECG
- using a nebulizer
- passing a urinary catheter
- controlling a haemorrhage and suturing a wound.

Although these skills may be assessed in a workplace-based setting, you could be presented in the CSA with a scenario that requires candidates, as part of the station, to demonstrate one of these skills on either a simulated patient or a manikin. Make sure you feel confident in being able to perform such tasks competently.

Further reading

Committee of General Practice Education Directors (COGPED). *Out of Hours (OOH) Training for GP Specialty Registrars* Revised Position Paper. London: COGPED, 2010

NHS Evidence Clinical Knowledge Summaries – Angina www.cks.nhs.uk/angina

NICE guidelines CG95 – Chest pain of recent onset. March 2010 http://guidance.nice.org.uk/CG95

RCGP curriculum statement 7 – Care of acutely ill people www.rcgp.org.uk (see Appendix 3: 'Dangerous' diagnoses)

Simon C, Everitt H, Van Dorp F, Schroeder K. *Oxford Handbook of General Practice* (3rd edn). Oxford: Oxford University Press, 2010

Thomas J, Monaghan T. *Oxford Handbook of Clinical Examination and Practical Skills*. Oxford: Oxford University Press, 2007

STATION 23

Information given to candidates

Marcus Harrison is a 58-year-old patient who rarely comes to the surgery.

His records show that he had a duodenal ulcer when he was 33 years old, for which he required surgery. He has not had any related symptoms since then.

As Marcus enters the consultation room you can see that he is not moving his right arm but has it flexed at the elbow and held against his body.

The first words the patient says when he enters the room are, 'Sorry to bother you, doctor, but my right shoulder has been giving me so much trouble, I can't sleep and driving my taxi is getting a real problem. I know that I shouldn't be taking the Brufen but it's the only thing that helps the pain. It's really starting to get me down.'

- What do you think this station is testing?
- Make notes or discuss your thoughts with a colleague before you read on.

Plan your approach to this station:

Information given to simulated patient

Basic details – You are Marcus Harrison, a 58-year-old taxi driver.

Appearance and behaviour – When you enter the consulting room you are holding your right arm against your body, with it bent at the elbow. If the doctor examines your shoulder there are no specific tender points but it feels generally sore. You find it painful to move your right arm at the shoulder in any direction, whether against resistance or not (i.e. forwards, backwards, outwards, or twisting the arm inwards or outwards), but you are able to do so by about 30 degrees in all directions (i.e. about a third of the way between having your arm by your side and having your elbow at the same height as your shoulder). The only exception to this is twisting or rotating the shoulder outwards – this is particularly painful and you cannot really manage it at all as the pain is so bad. You will not be able to put your right hand behind your head or place your right hand in the small of your back if asked to do so by the doctor. Your left shoulder is fine.

History

Freely divulged to doctor – You do not normally come to the doctor's but your right shoulder has been giving you problems for the last 4 weeks. It started off as a general ache with the joint feeling stiff. It has become increasingly painful, with restricted movement. You have been finding it hard to sleep as the pain wakes you up and is particularly bad if you lie on your right side. With the pain and not sleeping, things are really getting you down.

Divulged to doctor if specifically asked – You do not remember injuring or straining your shoulder. You feel the pain most in your upper outer arm, just below your shoulder joint. No other joints are affected. You have not noticed any swelling, heat or redness of your right shoulder. You have not had any neck pain. There is no tingling or numbness in your right arm or hand. You have been well in yourself otherwise and have not been feverish. You are right-handed, so the shoulder problem has been even more difficult to manage. You now brush your teeth and eat using your left hand. You have found it increasingly hard to work as your right shoulder has been so painful. You have been using your left arm to steer and try not to use your right arm, changing gears by taking your left hand off the steering wheel momentarily. Even getting dressed in the morning has become difficult, particularly if there are any front fastenings. You are not going to the toilet more frequently and you are not excessively thirsty.

Ideas, concerns and expectations – You think you may have strained your shoulder but you are not sure how you did this. You think it is best to rest your shoulder. You have heard from a friend that acupuncture can help shoulder pain and want to ask the doctor about this. A couple of your customers have commented on the way you take your hand off the steering wheel to change gears and you are worried that someone may report you. You know you should probably stop driving at the moment but you need the income. You are hoping the doctor will arrange an x-ray and may be able to offer you some treatment – some acupuncture or an injection.

First words spoken to doctor – 'Sorry to bother you, doctor, but my right shoulder has been giving me so much trouble, I can't sleep and driving my taxi is getting a real problem. I know that I shouldn't be taking the Brufen but it's the only thing that helps the pain. It's really starting to get me down.'

Medical history – You had an ulcer just beyond your stomach in your small bowel when you were 33 years old which required surgery. You have not had any further problems with ulcers since then. You are otherwise fit and well.

Drug history – You have been taking ibuprofen, which you bought at the supermarket, for the last 4 weeks. To start with you took only one or two 200 mg tablets a day. But as the shoulder pain worsened you started to take more and you are now taking two 200 mg tablets four times a day (which you know is more than the maximum it says on the packet). You did try paracetamol at first, but this did not seem to give much relief.

Social history – You work as a self-employed taxi driver. You have not smoked since you were a teenager. You used to drink heavily but after your ulcer surgery you stopped completely. You live with your wife and grown-up son.

Family history – There is no family history of diabetes or joint problems in your immediate family.

- Having read the information given to the simulated patient, what do you now think this station is testing?
- Make notes or discuss your thoughts with a colleague before you turn the page.

Review your approach to this station:

Tested at this station:

1. Generic communication skills.
2. History-taking skills.
3. Physical examination skills.
4. Reaching a shared management plan.

Domain 1 – Interpersonal skills

Generic communication skills

At each station in the Clinical Skills Assessment (CSA) you need to ensure that you demonstrate competence in all three domains (interpersonal skills; data gathering, technical and assessment skills; clinical management skills). At this station there is no specific communication issue, such as the patient being angry, talkative, or with a hearing or visual impairment. Indeed, the primary nature of this case is testing physical examination skills. However, you must still be able to demonstrate effective communication skills during the consultation, so the list below is a recap on some of these generic skills:

- Remember the importance of non-verbal communication, including body language and eye contact.
- Always start with open questions before moving on to more specific closed questions.
- Use paraphrasing, checking and summarizing to show that you are actively listening.
- Pick up on, and respond to, cues that the patient gives, such as his awareness that he should not be driving in his current condition.
- Always remember to ask about the patient's ideas, concerns and expectations. Does he have any thoughts about what is going on with his shoulder? Are there any particular concerns? What is he hoping will happen from coming to see you today?
- When giving information, such as explaining a diagnosis, avoid talking at length. Instead 'chunk and check', i.e. give information in manageable chunks, then check the patient's understanding before you move on.
- Avoid medical jargon and use lay terminology – appropriate to the patient – when explaining diagnosis and treatment options.
- Try to stay patient-centred during the consultation – in other words, identify the patient's agenda and address it.
- Give patients the opportunity to raise any other issues which they might not at first have mentioned – *'Is there anything else I can help you with today?'*
- Encourage patients to ask questions at the end of the consultation – *'What would you like to ask?'*
- Check understanding of the management plan, including follow-up. Can he say what the plan is that you have jointly agreed?

Domain 2 – Data gathering, technical and assessment skills

History-taking skills

When a patient presents with a painful joint you need to feel confident that you have excluded conditions requiring immediate action (e.g. septic arthritis or dislocation). You should also rule out other red flags that might prompt referral to a specialist. Next, you need to identify the likely structural origin of the pain (e.g. in this case neck, shoulder or elsewhere). Finally, if you feel the problem is indeed originating from the shoulder, you should try to differentiate between the common shoulder injuries (see Knowledge base). A focused history, together with examination, will help you do all this:

- He says his right shoulder has been giving him trouble. Can he say more about this?
- Where precisely is the pain: neck, shoulder or arm? Can he show you?
- Any history of trauma? Does the patient do any heavy exercise involving his arms?
- Is he well in himself otherwise – any fevers or general malaise?
- Any weight loss or problems with his breathing? Does he have pain at rest? Is there any history of cancer?
- Has his shoulder ever been dislocated? Does it feel unstable as though it might become dislocated?
- Has his shoulder swollen up? Has the skin over the joint been red or hot?
- Are any other joints affected?
- Has he had problems with his joints in the past?
- Is the pain worse first thing in the morning or later on in the day, or is there no pattern?
- Do any of the patient's immediate family suffer from joint problems (such as rheumatoid arthritis)?
- Any eye problems or pain passing urine (Reiter's syndrome)?
- Is the patient left- or right-handed?
- What effect has the shoulder problem had on his day-to-day life? He says that driving his taxi has become a real problem. Can he say more about how it is affecting his work?
- During the history you should also try to exclude referred angina or diaphragmatic irritation as causes of his shoulder pain.
- This patient has a history of peptic ulcer disease and he has been taking regular non-steroidal anti-inflammatory drugs (NSAIDs). You need to make sure that he has not experienced any symptoms suggesting recurrence of an ulcer or gastrointestinal bleed:
  - Any heartburn or indigestion recently?
  - Any abdominal pain?
  - Does he feel nauseous or has he vomited?
  - Has he seen any blood in his stools or have his stools changed colour such that they are now dark and tarry?

Physical examination skills

The GP curriculum lists examination of the shoulder as one of the psychomotor skills that you should be able competently to demonstrate. Indeed, physical examination is the 'nub' of this case. With any joint examination a rough guide is: look, feel, move (active, passive and against resistance):

- Explain the nature of the examination to the patient and gain consent.
- You can often pick up clues even before the start of the formal examination. This patient enters the room with his right arm immobile, flexed at the elbow and held against his body, which gives you an idea about his loss of function.
- Ask the patient to take his top off so you can examine the shoulder adequately. This also allows you to judge what gross movements he is able to perform.
- Inspection – both from in front and behind, look for signs of deformity, swelling, asymmetry, redness and muscle wasting.
- Palpation – palpate the sternoclavicular, acromioclavicular and glenohumeral joints, looking for signs of localized tenderness (see Knowledge base). The tendon of biceps is palpated anteriorly in the bicipital groove between the humeral greater and lesser tubercles.
- Assessing movement – as a quick screening test ask the patient to put his hands behind his head and then to place them in the small of his back. This is a gross test of a variety of movements at the shoulder joint, including flexion, extension, internal and external rotation.
- Assessing movement – active movement. In turn, ask the patient to flex, extend, abduct, adduct, externally and internally rotate the shoulder as far as he can. For abduction, you can fix the scapula to isolate glenohumeral joint function.
- Assessing movement – passive movement. If there are limitations of active movement, see whether you can passively move the joint beyond the limitations found on active movement. Frozen shoulder problems usually do not allow any further passive movement whereas rotator cuff injuries often do.
- Assessing movement – painful arc. Pain on abduction between 70° and 120° suggests rotator cuff injury, as does pain on abduction that is worse against resistance.
- Assess for crepitus during the examination.

There are no abnormalities on inspection apart from how the patient holds his right arm on entering the room. See Information given to simulated patient above for further positive findings.

Domain 3 – Clinical management skills

Reaching a shared management plan (overlap with domain 1)

This patient's history and examination findings suggest a glenohumeral joint disorder, namely frozen shoulder (adhesive capsulitis). However, mixed shoulder problems are common and the exact diagnostic category often does not change what is primarily conservative management in a general practice setting, namely analgesia, physiotherapy, and encouragement to return to normal activities as early as possible:

- Explain the probable diagnosis – how the capsule around the shoulder joint can become swollen and thickened and lead to pain and restricted movement.
- Give advice on prognosis – prepare the patient for a potentially protracted course, as symptoms can last for 2 or 3 years.
- Encourage self-management of his condition. Explain that keeping the shoulder mobile is a key goal. Gentle shoulder exercises several times a day will help. The exercises will involve some discomfort but are important to prevent muscle wasting.
- Pain management is a key element to facilitate mobilization and allow him to sleep better. You need to explain the risks associated with oral NSAIDs and negotiate their use. Has he thought about trying regular maximum-strength paracetamol, with a topical NSAID gel? He could then reserve oral ibuprofen for occasional use if the pain is particularly bad. You could also consider giving him a proton pump inhibitor – e.g. omeprazole 20 mg OD – for gastroprotection to cover his use of oral NSAIDs. Explain how he would need to discontinue NSAIDs if he started to suffer from indigestion.
- Offer the patient other treatment options, including steroid injections and physiotherapy. Physiotherapy will involve exercises and possibly heat treatment. Explain that the evidence for both treatments' long-term effectiveness is weak, but they may help with short-term relief. What does he think about these options?
- Explain that x-rays and blood tests are not indicated unless there are worrying (red flag) signs, and reassure him that he has none.
- Encourage early return to normal activities, if possible.
- However, at present it appears that his restricted movement renders him unsafe to drive. You should be explicit in your advice that he has a legal duty to inform the Driver and Vehicle Licensing Agency (DVLA) and must refrain from driving at this time. This advice has major implications for the patient and you need to explore his response sensitively and empathetically.
- He is reluctant to stop working due to financial pressures. You could offer to give him a 'Fit note' (Statement of Fitness for Work Med 3 form) as he may be entitled to Employment and Support Allowance (ESA) once he is off work through illness for 4 days or more.
- The patient wants to know about acupuncture treatment for his shoulder. You can advise him that there is little evidence to either confirm or refute the effectiveness of acupuncture for shoulder problems, but that it may improve pain and function for a few weeks.
- Frozen shoulder is five times more common in people with diabetes mellitus, but he has no symptoms and no family history so it is unlikely to need further investigation.

Knowledge base – Diagnosis of shoulder problems

Adapted with permission from Oxford Shoulder and Elbow Clinic shoulder diagnosis flowchart

Referral to a specialist is indicated if:

- red flags are present (see above)
- there is a history of joint instability
- there is significant disability and no improvement in pain over a 6-month period, despite conservative management
- there is diagnostic uncertainty.

Surgery may be considered if conservative treatment is unsuccessful.

> **Take-home messages**
> - Shoulder problems are common, can be protracted and mainly involve conservative management in primary care.
> - Always exclude red flags when patients present with joint pain.
> - Remember that at each CSA station you need to score marks in all three domains.

Tasks
- Re-run the scenario with the examination findings revealing a painful arc syndrome. Would this change the management options?
- Re-run the scenario with the patient refusing to stop driving.
- Re-run the scenario with the patient complaining of pain and swelling of the small joints of his hands.

1-minute explanations for patients
- Explain what painful arc syndrome is.
- Explain what would be involved with a steroid injection of the shoulder.
- Explain what exercises would be good to keep the shoulder mobile.

Ideas for further revision
Examination of a joint lends itself to inclusion in the CSA. Be sure that you have a good framework for examining the shoulder, knee, hip and back, and can apply the principles to any joint examination.

Further reading
GMC guidance – Confidentiality. Supplementary guidance: Reporting concerns about patients to the DVLA or DVA www.gmc-uk.org/guidance/ethical_guidance/confidentiality.asp

Lloyd M, Bor R. *Communication Skills for Medicine* (3rd edn). Edinburgh: Churchill Livingston, 2009

Murphy RJ, Carr AJ. Shoulder pain. Clinical evidence http://clinicalevidence.bmj.com. Web publication date 22 July 2010

NHS Evidence Clinical Knowledge Summaries – Frozen shoulder www.cks.nhs.uk

Thomas J, Monaghan T. *Oxford Handbook of Clinical Examination and Practical Skills*. Oxford: Oxford University Press, 2007

Information given to candidates

Fatima Ahmed is an Urdu speaker who rarely comes to the surgery. At previous appointments for minor illnesses family members have acted as interpreters.

She is 38 years old and married with three children.

She attended hospital 8 weeks ago to have a vulval cyst removed. The discharge letter from the gynaecology team states:

Dear GP,

Mrs Ahmed attended for a planned procedure under general anaesthetic to remove a vulval cyst. This went well and the histology shows no worrying findings. However, during the procedure there appeared to be a fistula in the posterior vaginal wall communicating with the rectum, which was discharging a small amount of pus into the vagina. It was felt that the fistula would probably close on its own. We discussed options with the patient and it was agreed to 'wait and see'. If things are no better in 4–6 weeks' time then please refer her back for further management.

When the patient enters the room she has a trained interpreter with her, Mrs Lone, who was booked by one of the receptionists.

- What do you think this station is testing?
- Make notes or discuss your thoughts with a colleague before you read on.

Plan your approach to this station:

Information given to simulated patient

Basic details – You are Fatima Ahmed, an Urdu speaker and 38-year-old mother of three, originally from Pakistan. You came to the UK when you were 34 years old to join your husband, who had moved here the year before. You are not able to speak much English at all, but you do understand simple spoken English quite well.

Appearance and behaviour – You are wearing a headscarf. You are softly spoken and do not make much eye contact. You answer the doctor's questions in a direct manner – through the interpreter – although at times you appear to be embarrassed at discussing these personal matters.

History

Freely divulged to doctor – You went to hospital about 2 months ago to have a cyst removed. Soon after leaving hospital you noticed a small amount of yellow discharge from your vagina which has occurred on and off since then. It has still not cleared up so you decided to visit the GP. Your husband is away on family business in Pakistan, so you came down to the surgery on your own.

Divulged to doctor if specifically asked – The doctors at the hospital told you that the procedure went well and that they would send the results to your GP, after looking at the cyst under a microscope. But you were also told that there appeared to be a 'channel' which should not have been there. You did not really understand what they meant or where the 'channel' was. You have not been feverish or felt unwell. You have never had any sexually transmitted infections. You had a healthy sex life with your husband before you attended the hospital but have not had intercourse since, due to the operation and the subsequent vaginal discharge. Apart from your husband, you have not had any other sexual partners since you were married 12 years ago. You have not had any pelvic or abdominal pain, or any pain on intercourse. Your periods are regular – the last one was 2 weeks ago. You have been opening your bowels and passing urine without any problems. You have not felt down or depressed recently.

Ideas, concerns and expectations – You had noticed the cyst several months ago and had been glad to have the operation to get rid of it. When you were in hospital it was difficult to fully understand the doctors as they used long words. But one of the nurses spoke Urdu and would come and see you to explain what the doctors had said. But this nurse was not around when you were told about the 'channel'. You are worried that the discharge has not cleared up. You are hoping the doctor today will explain what the 'channel' is and where the discharge is coming from, and refer you back to the hospital.

First words spoken to doctor – 'I have come to the doctor's as I still have a discharge.'

Medical history – You attended hospital in Pakistan for your first child's birth, but since then have not been back in a hospital until the removal of the cyst on your vulva (the external parts of the female genitals) 2 months ago. All three births have been uncomplicated vaginal deliveries. You are otherwise fit and well.

Drug history – You had 2 weeks' supply of antibiotics after you left hospital 2 months ago. You do not take any regular medication. As far as you know you are not allergic to any medication.

Social history — You live with your husband and three children — all girls under 10. You were fairly well educated in Pakistan, although your spoken English has always been poor. You work as a counsellor at the local Pakistani community support centre 3 days a week. Your extended family lives nearby and offers a great deal of support, including childcare. You have a good circle of friends that are all from the local Urdu-speaking community. Your husband has his own wholesale business which he runs with two of his cousins. You do not drink alcohol or smoke.

Family history — There are no major illnesses in your immediate family.

Information given to simulated interpreter

Basic details — You are Mrs Lone, a 55-year-old professional interpreter who speaks Urdu. You live in another city, 20 miles away. You have just met the patient for the first time in the waiting room.

Appearance and behaviour — You are professionally dressed and solely interpret the doctor's questions and the patient's responses.

- Having read the information given to the simulated patient and interpreter, what do you now think this station is testing?
- Make notes or discuss your thoughts with a colleague before you turn the page.

Review your approach to this station:

Tested at this station:

1. Conducting a consultation using an interpreter.
2. History-taking skills.
3. Physical examination.
4. Negotiating a shared management plan.

Domain 1 – Interpersonal skills

Conducting a consultation using an interpreter

Ideally, an interpreter should be as unobtrusive as possible. However, the consultation dynamic will undoubtedly change significantly. You need to try to minimize this effect as much as possible:

- Set up the seating arrangement in a triangle, with both yourself and the patient able to see the interpreter.
- Introduce yourself and the interpreter to the patient.
- Explain what the role of the interpreter will be during the consultation and reassure the patient that what is discussed is confidential, for both yourself and the interpreter.
- At the start, tell the interpreter to ask for clarification from you if she does not fully understand what you are asking her to translate.
- Speak directly to the patient, observe her reactions and maintain eye contact to allow you to respond with non-verbal recognition to the interpreter's translation (e.g. head nods, smiles).
- Use the second person when conducting the interview, i.e. 'What do *you* think about *your* problem?' rather than 'What does *she* think about *her* problem?' This encourages you to have a conversation with the patient rather than with the interpreter.
- Use unambiguous words and avoid medical jargon.
- Be alert to whether the interpreter appears to be answering for the patient rather than translating what is said. This is less likely with a trained interpreter.
- Be aware that if the interpreter is from the same local community as the patient, it may be difficult for the patient to speak openly.

Domain 2 – Data gathering, technical and assessment skills

History-taking skills

You need to use the skills outlined above while taking a comprehensive history of the patient's complaint:

- Open questions and exploration of the patient's ideas, concerns and expectations should help you understand her perspective on events.
- Acknowledge that it can be difficult talking about these matters, but that it is important to try to understand about the discharge.
- More specific closed questions will allow you to obtain details about her current symptoms:
  - What is the discharge like? Does she have to wear pads?
  - Is the discharge there all the time or does it come and go?

- Any fever or weight loss, or lack of appetite?
- Any pain in her tummy, or lower down at the front?
- Any back pain?
- Any pain during sexual intercourse?
- When was her last period – any different from usual? Any inter-menstrual or post-coital bleeding?
- Any problems when she opens her bowels? Or urinates?
- Has she ever had any sexually transmitted infections?
- Has she ever suffered from any other medical problems? Any previous operations? Any problems with previous deliveries?
- Any family history of bowel problems?

- Vaginal discharge should usually prompt you to take a full sexual history. However, in this case, as you already know about the fistula you may feel this is not necessary.

Physical examination

Time is particularly short at this station since all dialogue needs to be translated by the interpreter. The examiner will intervene if you start to mention physical examination and tell you to assume that you have conducted a full abdominal and pelvic examination, including swabs, and that the findings are normal apart from a small amount of yellow discharge seen in the vagina.

Domain 3 – Clinical management skills

Negotiating a shared management plan

The key management action point for this station is to offer to refer the patient back to the hospital team for further investigation of her fistula. However, you also need to explain to the patient about the fistula findings:

- The patient is embarrassed at the personal nature of the discussion. You should be alert to this and recognize that her embarrassment may be increased by cultural or social influences.
- She has asked about the histology results for the removed cyst. You can reassure her that these are fine.
- Explaining the fistula findings may be more easily done by drawing a simple diagram.
- You should be honest and explain that you are not sure why the fistula is there, but that, if she would like you to, you could ask the hospital team to see her again to investigate this further.
- When explaining the problem and management options, ask her to repeat back what has been said, to check understanding.
- Repeatedly encourage the patient to ask questions.
- Would it be useful if someone came with her to her next appointment, to offer support?
- If possible, could the interpreter liaise with the patient to ensure that the same interpreter is present at any future appointments with the hospital doctors?

Knowledge base – Interviewing with an interpreter

Key points

- Address the patient in the second person.
- Talk directly to the patient.
- Keep control of the consultation.
- Pause frequently.
- Appear attentive when patient responds.
- Respond to non-verbal cues.
- Check the patient's understanding.
- Make use of written material.

Further points

- Ensure that you make clear to the interpreter that you wish them to translate your words verbatim and similarly interpret the patient's answers verbatim, rather than the interpreter speaking on behalf of the patient.
- If you know that an interpreter will be present, try to book a longer appointment.
- Be aware that some primary care organizations have contracts with language lines, where interpreters are available 24 hours a day, via the telephone, in most languages.
- At the end of the consultation you could ask the interpreter for feedback on the communication issues. Could you have made the interpreter's job easier?

> **Take-home messages**
>
> - When conducting consultations using an interpreter, try to build rapport using the physical set-up of the room, good eye contact and non-verbal responses.
> - Allow patients using interpreters repeated opportunities to ask questions and seek clarification.
> - Drawing explanatory diagrams is often useful.

Tasks

- Re-run the scenario with the interpreter being one of the patient's teenage daughters. How might this change how you managed the consultation?
- Re-run the scenario with the interpreter repeatedly speaking on behalf of the patient rather than interpreting. How might you manage this?
- Re-run the scenario with the interpreter being via a telephone (e.g. Language Line).

1-minute explanations for patients

- Explain what a recto-vaginal fistula is.
- Explain what might be the options for management of the fistula.
- Explain why it is important to consider definitive treatment for the fistula.

Ideas for further revision

The GP curriculum states that one of the learning objectives for trainees is to develop communication skills including working with interpreters to deal with patients from diverse backgrounds. If you work in an ethnically diverse area then you should have ample opportunity to practise these skills. If not, you could ask your programme director to arrange teaching sessions with simulated patients and interpreters. You could also contact trained interpreters working in healthcare settings where translation services are required, to try to understand the various issues that arise within these consultations.

Further reading

Adams K. Making the best use of health advocates and interpreters. *BMJ Career Focus* 2002; 325 http://careers.bmj.com

Phelan M, Parkman S. How to Do It: Work with an interpreter. *BMJ* 1995; 311: 555–557 www.bmj.com

RCGP curriculum statement 3.4 – Promoting equality and valuing diversity www.rcgp.org.uk

RCGP curriculum statement 10.1 – Women's health www.rcgp.org.uk

Roberts C, Moss B, Wass V, Sarangi S, Jones R. Misunderstandings: a qualitative study of primary care consultations in multilingual settings, and educational implications. *Medical Education* 2005; 39 (5): 465–475

Information given to candidates

Tony Barrett is a 58-year-old patient who rarely visits the surgery.

He was seen 7 days ago by your colleague with a subconjunctival haemorrhage in his left eye. There was no pain or any visual problems reported by the patient at that time.

Full examination of his eyes, including acuity, fundoscopy, eye movements and pupillary response, were all normal. His blood pressure (BP) was 128/82 mmHg.

His records state that he had asked whether he needed to take time off work for his subconjunctival haemorrhage and that your colleague advised him this was not necessary.

You note that he was seen on two occasions 4 months ago with a bad back, which gradually resolved with symptomatic relief and physiotherapy. He received sick notes (Statement of Fitness for Work) for a total of 6 weeks during that episode.

As the patient enters the consultation room he says, 'All I need is a sick note for my eye for last week, but I don't understand why I've been waiting 40 bloody minutes.'

If you decide to examine the patient today, assume that BP is normal and there is no abnormality of either eye.

- What do you think this station is testing?
- Make notes or discuss your thoughts with a colleague before you read on.

Plan your approach to this station:

Information given to simulated patient

Basic details – You are Tony Barrett, a 58-year-old single man who works as a fork-lift truck driver.

Appearance and behaviour – You are angry at having to wait 40 minutes to see the doctor today. However, if the doctor is understanding and apologetic you will soon calm down and even apologize for being 'a bit rude' when you came in.

History

Freely divulged to doctor – You woke up last week with what looked like blood in your left eye. Nothing like that had ever happened to you before so you booked an emergency appointment to see the doctor. She checked you over and told you it was 'a bleed into the eye'. You were due to work two night shifts starting that night, but when you got home you thought it would be best to take it easy and called in sick. You went back to work after missing those two night shifts as the eye seemed to be improving. Now your work wants a doctor's sick note to cover the time you were off.

Divulged to doctor if specifically asked – You have not had any pain or problems with your vision in either eye. You remember the other doctor saying you did not need to take any time off work, but after you had walked home you thought that 'to be on the safe side' you should stay at home. The red patch of blood in your left eye gradually disappeared over the following week. You have never had anything go into your eyes and your work is not an environment where this happens. You have not suffered from any headaches.

Ideas, concerns and expectations – Although you felt that the doctor checked you over thoroughly last week, you were worried when she said that you had 'a bleed into the eye' and did not quite understand the diagnosis. Four months ago you took 6 weeks off work with a bad back and had to see the sickness manager about this. You felt under pressure to return to work then, and you were told that he would be keeping an eye on your sick leave. You are afraid that work may target you for redundancy because of your time off and you think having a doctor's certificate will help matters. You believe that you are entitled to a sick note even if you have taken only two night shifts off, as you think things looked pretty bad in your eye last week. Initially you will not be happy if the doctor says he cannot give you a standard sick note, but if the doctor acknowledges your worries about work and clearly explains the situation regarding issuing a retrospective sick note, you will accept this. As a compromise, you would be prepared to pay for a private sick note if the doctor offers this as an option.

First words spoken to doctor – 'All I need is a sick note for my eye for last week, but I don't understand why I've been waiting 40 bloody minutes.'

Medical history – You strained your back 4 months ago and were off work for 6 weeks. You took pain killers and saw a physiotherapist privately, which helped considerably, and you have not had any problems since going back to work. You are otherwise fit and well.

Drug history – You do not take any regular medication and have no drug allergies.

Social history – You live on your own. You have never been married but have a close group of friends from work and the local brass band, of which you have been a member since you were 12 years old. You do shift work in an engineering plant, mostly using a fork-lift truck to stack the metal sheet products that your company produces. You stopped smoking when you were 24 years old and drink one or two pints of beer on Friday and Saturday nights.

Family history – There are no major health problems in your family. As far as you know, no one in your family has had glaucoma or any eye problems other than wearing glasses for reading.

- Having read the information given to the simulated patient, what do you now think this station is testing?
- Make notes or discuss your thoughts with a colleague before you turn the page.

Review your approach to this station:

Tested at this station:

1. Dealing with an angry patient.
2. History-taking skills.
3. Physical examination.
4. Dealing with a sick note request.

Domain 1 – Interpersonal skills

Dealing with an angry patient

Dealing with patients' emotions is a key skill which can be readily tested in the Clinical Skills Assessment (CSA):

- This patient is angry at being kept waiting 40 minutes. As a first step, acknowledge his anger and make a sincere apology for the delay.
- Avoid the temptation to blame someone or something else for the delay, e.g. 'I'm sorry but the receptionist keeps making mistakes with our new booking system.'
- Apologizing – repeatedly if necessary – demonstrates that you are prepared to take responsibility for the delay rather than sidestepping or dismissing it.
- If he continues to be angry, ask whether there is anything else upsetting him today.
- Be aware of your emotional response to such situations. You may feel under attack and angry with the patient for taking his frustrations out on you. You need to have strategies for dealing with these emotions to allow you to remain professional and patient-centred during the consultation.
- Avoid responses to angry patients that can lead to further confrontation or an escalation of the situation, e.g. being defensive or contradictory ('Well, the computer shows that you arrived late, so have only been waiting 30 minutes.').
- You will have some difficult negotiating to do regarding the sick note request later on in the consultation, so it is all the more important to fully address, and defuse, the patient's anger at the start.
- If at any time you feel threatened or physically intimidated by an angry patient, you should end the consultation and remove yourself from the room.

Domain 2 – Data gathering, technical and assessment skills

History-taking skills

Once the patient has calmed down, you need to take a history to see whether there have been any developments since your colleague saw him last week. You also need to explore his understanding and any concerns he may have about his eye:

- He wants a sick note to cover him for last week. For your benefit, could he recap why he came to see the doctor then?
- What is his understanding of the problem with his eye last week?
- Since then has he experienced any new symptoms, including:
  - headaches
  - visual problems (e.g. double vision, blurred vision)
  - eye pain

- soreness or irritation
- a sensation that there is something in his eye?
- Is there any history of anything going into his eye, e.g. at work?
- How have things progressed with the blood he saw in the white of his eye last week?
- This patient was worried last week when he heard that he had 'a bleed into the eye'. Was there anything he was particularly worried about? Does he understand that although it may have looked dramatic, the condition is not serious?

Physical examination

His records state that when your colleague examined the patient last week there was nothing to find except a subconjunctival haemorrhage in his left eye. You are told that today there is no abnormality of either eye and that his BP is normal.

Domain 3 – Clinical management skills

Dealing with a sick note request

The patient wants a sick note for last week, even though your colleague advised him that he did not need to take any time off work. Trying to understand why he wants a sick note will help you address his concerns and help you to negotiate an outcome that is acceptable to both of you:

- Why does he feel he needs a sick note for last week?
- Has his employer asked him to obtain one?
- Is he concerned that having time off without a sick note will affect how he is treated at work?
- Has he had much time off work recently through illness?
- Did he discuss obtaining a sick note when he saw the doctor last week?
- You can advise him that employers should not routinely ask for a doctor's sick note for the first 7 days of an illness, as employees are able to self-certify for this period.
- However, the patient appears not to have fully understood the diagnosis last week and was concerned about 'a bleed into the eye', so one option would be to offer to write a private sick note. Does he realize that this will incur a fee? What does he think about this as a way forward?
- You may be reluctant to issue any type of sick note if you think this would undermine your colleague. However, there has clearly been some misunderstanding in that the patient genuinely felt that his problem was significant.
- In this scenario there is no one right answer on how to deal with the request for a sick note, but a good candidate would fully explore the patient's concerns, make sure that he understood the nature of the diagnosis, and empathetically explain the situation and options regarding the issuing of sick notes in this case.

Knowledge base – Issuing sick notes

Reference: Department for Work and Pensions guidance on Statement of Fitness for Work, 2010.

Statement of Fitness for Work (Med 3)	'Fit notes' differ from previous forms in that: • telephone consultations are now an acceptable form of assessment • option of 'May be fit for work' • in first 6 months of sickness, Statements can be issued for no longer than 3 months • there is one form to issue Statements prospectively and retrospectively • more space for comments on the functional effect of the patient's condition • removal of the option to say a patient is fit for work.
Who can issue a Statement of Fitness for Work?	• Can only be completed by a doctor. • However, a doctor can base their decision on a written report from another doctor or registered healthcare professional.
What if a patient asks for a 'fit for work' Statement?	• It is a common myth that employees are required to be 'signed back to work'. This is not the case in most situations. Where required there is an existing procedure (e.g. Driver and Vehicle Licensing Agency (DVLA) Form D4 for Group 2 drivers). • If an employer feels they require such advice they can seek this from a GP or occupational health specialist via a private arrangement.
Why a move from 'sick note' to 'fit note'?	• Clear evidence of the therapeutic nature of work to promote recovery and rehabilitation. • Risk of 'worklessness' state if off work for protracted period. • Much sickness absence is due to mild/moderate mental ill health or musculoskeletal or cardiorespiratory conditions, which can often be accommodated for at work.

- After the first 6 months of incapacity, a Statement can be issued for any clinically appropriate period up to 'an indefinite period'.

Take-home messages

- You need to feel confident managing an angry patient both in everyday practice and in an exam setting such as the Clinical Skills Assessment (CSA).
- Acknowledging the patient's anger and apologizing can help diffuse the situation and allow you to move on to address their presenting complaint.
- Doctors need to work within the statutory framework governing the issuing of sick notes.

Tasks

- Re-run the scenario with the patient having been off work for 2 weeks with a bad back and now asking for a 'fit for work' note.
- Re-run the scenario with the patient asking for a note for his employer to say that he had attended the surgery the previous week.
- Re-run the scenario with the patient having been off work for 2 weeks with a bad back having not seen any health professional regarding this, and now wanting a sick note to cover the second week off work.

- You may want to re-run some of the other scenarios in the book with the patient initially presenting as angry, to practise your skills at defusing such situations in a variety of contexts.

1-minute explanations for patients

- Explain what a subconjunctival haemorrhage is.
- Explain why it is important to try to avoid being off work sick for extended periods, if possible.
- Explain the implications if you tick the 'May be fit for work' box on the form.

Ideas for further revision

In the CSA you might have to deal with patients displaying a range of challenging emotions or behaviours. Think about, and practise with colleagues, how you would approach patients presenting with distress, anger, a dismissive attitude, reticence or over-familiarity.

Further reading

Department for Work and Pensions. Statement of Fitness for Work – A guide for general practitioners and other doctors. February 2010 www.dwp.gov.uk/docs/fitnote-gp-guide.pdf

Maguire P. *Communication Skills for Doctors*. London: Arnold, 2000

Warning – readers may find some of the language used in this station offensive.

Information given to candidates

Jim Nelson is a 38-year-old obese patient who suffers from hypertension.

He has been taking amlodipine 5 mg OD for the last 6 months.

When he saw the nurse for a blood pressure (BP) check 2 weeks ago it was 138/80 mmHg.

His body mass index (BMI) was found to be 34 kg/m^2.

His records state that he is a smoker.

The first thing the patient says when he enters the room is, 'Doctor, I need something stronger for my indigestion. I had a large Chinky meal last week and that set it off, and the other day after eating a samosa from the Paki shop things were really bad.'

- What do you think this station is testing?
- Make notes or discuss your thoughts with a colleague before you read on.

Plan your approach to this station:

Information given to simulated patient

Basic details – You are Jim Nelson, a 38-year-old single man, originally from Glasgow.

Appearance and behaviour – You are overweight. If the doctor challenges you about the language you use in your opening statement, initially you will be surprised – you did not think that such words would cause offence. So long as the doctor is polite and does not go on at length about what you have said, you will apologize and say that you will try not to use such words again. Overall, you will not be too bothered by the doctor's comments about your language – you really just want to get your indigestion sorted out.

History

Freely divulged to doctor – You have had intermittent heartburn for about 5 years now. Things have been worse in the last 3 or 4 months. Last year you only had problems only two or three times a month, whereas now you are getting symptoms three or four times a week. You feel an uncomfortable sensation in your upper abdomen and behind your breastbone, usually after meals. Lying down makes things worse. You have never been to the doctor's about your indigestion before. You are otherwise well.

Divulged to doctor if specifically asked – In the past, your symptoms settled with antacid tablets suggested by your local pharmacist; however, recently they do not seem to help as much. Things are worse after large meals and at night. You have not felt nauseous or vomited. You have no problems swallowing. You have never seen any blood when you open your bowels. Your stools have not been darker or black. Your appetite is fine and you have not lost any weight. Your pain never radiates into your arms and you do not experience any pain when you exert yourself, such as climbing a flight of stairs. You do not suffer from shortness of breath. You have not had any time off work due to your symptoms. You do not feel particularly stressed at the moment.

Ideas, concerns and expectations – When you first speak to the doctor you do not mean to upset or insult anyone by your choice of words, but are just trying to describe where and when the indigestion was particularly bad. Where you grew up in Glasgow everyone used these terms without people commenting. You are not concerned that your indigestion is anything serious, but it is worse now and the symptoms are really unpleasant. You know that you should probably cut out spicy foods. You are hoping the doctor can prescribe something to help.

First words spoken to doctor – 'Doctor, I need something stronger for my indigestion. I had a large Chinky meal last week and that set it off, and the other day after eating a samosa from the Paki shop things were really bad.'

Medical history – You were told that you had high BP 6 months ago, after it was checked by the doctor and nurse several times. But the tablets seem to be working and the nurse was happy with your BP when you had it checked a couple of weeks ago.

Drug history – You have been taking one tablet in the morning for your BP – amlodipine 5 mg – for the last 6 months. You have been taking antacids, such as Rennies®, for about 5 years, although you are using them more frequently now. You are not allergic to any medication.

Social history – You work shifts in the local meat-packing factory. You smoke 20 cigarettes a day and drink a couple of pints most nights when you are not working. Your brother is a member of the British National Party (BNP, a right-wing political party advocating resettlement of immigrants living in Britain back to their 'lands of ethnic origin'). You are not a BNP member but you are sympathetic to some of their views on immigration. You live with your brother on an almost exclusively white council estate.

Family history – There is no history of serious medical problems in your immediate family.

- Having read the information given to the simulated patient, what do you now think this station is testing?
- Make notes or discuss your thoughts with a colleague before you turn the page.

Review your approach to this station:

Tested at this station:

1. Understanding of equality and diversity issues: challenging a patient's racist language.
2. History-taking skills.
3. Physical examination.
4. Reaching a shared management plan.

Domain 1 – Interpersonal skills

Understanding of equality and diversity issues: challenging a patient's racist language

This is a particularly sensitive and difficult station. The patient has used words that are derogatory and offensive. 'Chinky' is considered an ethnic slur for Chinese people and 'Paki' has pejorative connotations and is used as a term of abuse towards those from the Indian sub-continent. As such, this language, even when describing food or shops rather than people, is indirect racist comment and therefore unacceptable:

- It would be easy to ignore the patient's terminology and focus on his physical complaint. However, doing so would be an abdication of your responsibility to promote equality and diversity and to challenge discriminatory language.
- The GP curriculum states that issues of equality and diversity are at the heart of the work of GPs and that you should recognize, respect, value and harness difference. Indeed, the curriculum learning outcomes say that a GP should be able to challenge behaviour that infringes the rights of others and recognize and take action to address discrimination.
- Although this patient does not mean to cause offence by his remarks, to ignore his use of these derogatory terms could be interpreted as tacit acceptance of his inappropriate language.
- The doctor–patient relationship is usually one based on trust and involves a duty of care on the doctor towards the patient. This can make it difficult to confront patients over inappropriate or offensive behaviour or language. However, as healthcare professionals we need to uphold high standards and to ensure that the environment we work in is free from discriminatory terminology or practices.
- You can allow him to finish his opening narrative, then explain that the words he has used are considered offensive and ask him not to use them again.
- How you deliver this comment is key – be polite but clear in your request. For example, *'Some people find the words you use to describe the Chinese meal and the shop run by British Asians offensive. Can I ask you not to repeat them? Thank you.'*
- If the patient responds in a hostile way, you will need to deal with his anger before moving on.
- When possible, move the patient on by asking about his physical complaint, demonstrating a caring and professional consulting style, and treating him in just the same way as you would any other patient.

Domain 2 – Data gathering, technical and assessment skills

History-taking skills

You need to take an appropriate history to exclude red flags and to try to understand the impact of the patient's symptoms on his daily life:

- He says his indigestion has got worse recently. Can he say more about this?
- How long has he suffered from this problem?
- Can he tell you more about his indigestion. What does it feel like? Does he ever get the sensation of acid coming up into his mouth? Is it worse lying down?
- Where exactly does he feel the discomfort? Does it radiate anywhere, e.g. through to his back or into his arms?
- How bad have things been at their worst?
- He says that take-away foods make things worse. Does anything else bring on his indigestion? What helps relieve his symptoms?
- Does he have the discomfort constantly or intermittently? What are things like at night?
- Has he felt nauseous or vomited?
- Any bleeding from his back passage? Have his stools become darker or appeared tarry black?
- Has he lost any weight recently? What is his appetite like?
- Any difficulty swallowing?
- Any chest pain when he exerts himself? Does he ever get short of breath with the pain?
- Does he smoke? How much alcohol does he drink?
- What sort of impact are his symptoms having on his day-to-day life? Has he had to take time off work due to his problem?
- Has he been under particular stress recently?
- You know that he is prescribed amlodipine for hypertension. Does he use this regularly and does he take any other medication, including over-the-counter drugs, such as ibuprofen? See knowledge base below for information on drugs that can cause dyspepsia.
- What does he think is going on with his worsening symptoms? What is he hoping will come from seeing you today?

Physical examination

This is a fairly full station, with candidates needing to cover the issues around the patient's language, his presentation with dyspepsia, and management of his symptoms, including lifestyle advice, all in 10 minutes. You should say that you would like to examine his abdomen, but you will be told the findings and not be required to actually perform the examination:

The only positive findings on abdominal examination are obesity and mild tenderness on deep palpation of the epigastrium.

Domain 3 – Clinical management skills

Reaching a shared management plan (overlap with domain 1)

This patient's diagnosis is uninvestigated dyspepsia with no red-flag symptoms or signs. Given his age, the history and examination findings there is currently no indication for endoscopy (see Knowledge base). If you decide to prescribe for dyspepsia, note that the GP curriculum states that you should be able to demonstrate a consistent and evidence-based approach:

- Reassure the patient that his symptoms are common and that there are no worrying signs.
- Empathize with him that dyspepsia can be very unpleasant and that you understand how it is now significantly affecting his quality of life.
- Explain that lifestyle changes could help his symptoms considerably, including:
  - stopping smoking
  - cutting down on alcohol
  - losing weight.
- What small steps might he realistically be able to take to start to make these changes?
- Other measures that he may find helpful include:
  - raising the head of his bed
  - avoiding eating late in the evening
  - cutting down on spicy and fatty foods
  - cutting down on caffeine and chocolate.
- Discuss how the medication he takes for his BP might be making his symptoms worse, and that one option is to change to another tablet. What does he think about this?
- Other options which you could discuss with him include:
  - empirical treatment with a proton pump inhibitor (PPI) for 1 month, e.g. omeprazole 20 mg OD or lansoprazole 30 mg OD
  - testing for *Helicobacter pylori* – using either urea breath test or stool antigen test, and treating if appropriate.
- The National Institute for Health and Clinical Excellence (NICE) states that there is no strong evidence as to which of the above two options (trial of a PPI or *Helicobacter pylori* test and treat) should be tried first. However, the patient is keen for you to prescribe him something to help with his symptoms, so a trial of a PPI with a review in a month might be the most appropriate option, so long as you make it clear that this should be in addition to lifestyle changes.
- Explain that if the trial of a PPI together with lifestyle changes helps to control his symptoms, he should try to return to self-treatment with antacid and/or alginate therapy (e.g. Gaviscon®), as required.
- Make sure you safety-net appropriately. Explain that the patient should seek immediate medical help if he experiences any signs or symptoms suggesting a perforation or gastrointestinal bleed.

Knowledge base

National Institute for Clinical Excellence (NICE) (2004) CG 17 Dyspepsia – management of dyspepsia in adults in primary care (Quick Reference Guide) London: NICE. Available from www.nice.org.uk/CG017. Reproduced with permission.

New episode of dyspepsia

| Entry or final state |
| Action |
| Action and outcome |

No ← Referral criteria met?[1] → **Yes**

Suspend Non-steroidal anti-inflammatory drug (NSAID) use and review medication[2]

Upper gastrointestinal (GI) malignancy

NUD — Endoscopy findings?

GORD   PUD

Treat uninvestigated dyspepsia

Treat non-ulcer dyspepsia (NUD)

Treat gastro-oesophageal reflux disease (GORD)

Treat peptic ulcer disease (PUD)

Review → Return to self-care

Refer to specialist

1. Immediate referral is indicated for significant acute GI bleeding. Consider the possibility of cardiac or biliary disease as part of the differential diagnosis. Urgent specialist referral (i.e. within 2 weeks) for endoscopic investigation is indicated for patients of any age with dyspepsia when presenting with any of the following: chronic gastrointestinal bleeding, progressive unintentional weight loss, progressive difficulty swallowing, persistent vomiting, iron-deficiency anaemia, epigastric mass or suspicious barium meal. Routine endoscopic investigation of patients of any age, presenting with dyspepsia and without alarm signs, is not necessary. However, in patients aged 55 years and older with unexplained*and persistent† recent-onset dyspepsia alone, an urgent referral for endoscopy should be made.
2. Review medications for possible causes of dyspepsia, for example calcium antagonists, nitrates, theophyllines, bisphosphonates, steroids and NSAIDs. Patients undergoing endoscopy should be free from medication with either a PPI or an H2 receptor antagonist for a minimum of 2 weeks.

   *See NICE guidelines for full definition of 'unexplained'. Can be taken to mean that common precipitants, such as NSAIDs, have been excluded.
   †See NICE guidelines for full definition of 'persistent'. Can be taken to mean up to 4–6 weeks, depending on the signs and symptoms.

Take-home messages

- We all have a duty to challenge discriminatory language or behaviour by patients or colleagues.
- Endoscopy is not routinely indicated for patients presenting with dyspepsia.
- The management of uninvestigated dyspepsia in primary care includes modifying exacerbating factors, lifestyle advice, trial of a PPI and *H. pylori* testing.

Tasks

- Re-run the scenario with the patient wearing an offensive T-shirt rather than saying anything offensive. Would you handle this any differently?
- Re-run the scenario with the patient starting by saying that they are glad that they were able to see a white doctor.
- Re-run the scenario with the patient continuing to use offensive language during the consultation. How would you manage this?

1-minute explanations for patients

- Explain what happens when patients experience dyspepsia.
- Explain what 'acid reflux' is.
- Explain what is involved in having an upper GI endoscopy.

Ideas for further revision

Try role-playing with colleagues what you would say to patients who made derogatory comments about another GP at your practice, swore at you during the consultation, or made sexually inappropriate comments about one of the reception staff.

Further reading

Chiba N. Managing uninvestigated dyspepsia in primary care. *BMJ* 2008; 336: 623 www.bmj.com

MeReC Briefing: The management of dyspepsia in primary care. March 2005; 32: 1–8 www.npc.nhs.uk/merec/therap/dysp/resources/merec_bulletin_vol16_no3.pdf

NHS Evidence Clinical Knowledge Summaries. Dyspepsia. www.cks.nhs.uk

NICE guidelines – Dyspepsia – management of dyspepsia in adults in primary care. August 2004 (amended June 2005) www.nice.org.uk

RCGP curriculum statement 15.2 – Clinical management: digestive problems www.rcgp.org.uk.

Information given to candidates

Mary French is a 48-year-old patient who suffers from hypertension.

Her blood pressure (BP) has been well controlled, with the most recent readings being:

128/82 mmHg – last week

126/76 mmHg – last month

132/78 mmHg – 6 months ago

She has been taking lisinopril 10 mg OD for 3 years without any problems.

Cervical smears – up to date and normal.

Height – 152 cm; weight – 53 kg; body mass index (BMI) – 23 kg/m^2

Her records show that she is a nurse who works in the local gynaecology outpatient department.

Recent blood test results which the patient asked a colleague to take at work:

Full blood count (FBC)	Normal	Glucose	Normal
Ures and electrolytes (U&Es)	Normal	Total cholesterol	3.0 mmol/L
Liver function tests (LFTs)	Normal	High-density lipoprotein	1.6 mmol/L
Thyroid function tests (TFTs)	Normal	Low-density lipoprotein	1.4 mmol/L
Follicle-stimulating hormone (FSH)	40 IU/L		
Luteinizing hormone (LH)	20 IU/L		

As the patient enters the room she says, 'Doctor, I think I'm going through the change and I really need something for my hot flushes and sweats. I know that there's an increased risk of breast cancer, DVTs and PEs, but do you think HRT would help?'

- What do you think this station is testing?
- Make notes or discuss your thoughts with a colleague before you read on.

Plan your approach to this station:

Information given to simulated patient

Basic details – You are Mary French, a 48-year-old nurse.

Appearance and behaviour – You come across as confident and fairly knowledgeable about hormone replacement therapy (HRT). You occasionally use medical jargon such as 'perimenopausal' (meaning around the time of the menopause) and 'PE' (pulmonary embolism – a blood clot on the lung).

History

Freely divulged to doctor – Your periods used to be 'like clockwork' but over the last 9 months they have become more and more irregular. You now have a period every 2–3 months. You have been suffering from worsening hot flushes and night sweats for the last 12 months. These really bother you, particularly at work and in the summer. You know about HRT through your work, and you also had an informal chat with one of the gynaecology doctors about whether you should start HRT. She talked about some of the risks and benefits but said you should discuss things with your GP. You have read that there is a 50% increased risk of breast cancer with HRT and want to discuss this with the doctor.

Divulged to doctor if specifically asked – You or your immediate family have never had any problems with clots in your limbs or lungs. You do not suffer from varicose veins. You have never had any gynaecological problems or operations. You do not have migraines or diabetes. You have never had any heart problems and the nurse said that your recent cholesterol test was 'very good'. Your great-aunt was diagnosed with breast cancer when she was in her 80s, but died of a stroke soon after. You used to have a coil fitted for contraception but for the last 5 years have been using condoms with your husband. You have not experienced any problems with vaginal dryness or urinary symptoms. Your mood has been fine.

Ideas, concerns and expectations – You are aware of the 'media scares' about HRT being associated with breast cancer and blood clots and, despite your work, you still feel a little anxious about starting HRT. In particular, you are concerned that your great-aunt had breast cancer, and that you used to smoke and now have tablets for BP. You are unsure to what degree these factors could further increase the risks of taking HRT. From the knowledge you have already, and because your symptoms are so unpleasant, you have rationalized that you should probably try HRT, but you want the doctor to go over the risks and hopefully reassure you that these are small. Your friend has HRT patches and you know how to use these. If you decide to start HRT, you would like to try patches first. You also want to know what the doctor thinks about herbal alternatives.

First words spoken to doctor – 'Doctor, I think I'm going through the change and I really need something for my hot flushes and sweats. I know that there's an increased risk of breast cancer, DVTs and PEs, but do you think HRT would help?'

Medical history – You were diagnosed with high BP 3 years ago and this has been well controlled with medication.

Drug history – You take one lisinopril 10 mg tablet every morning. You are not allergic to any medication.

Social history – You work at the local hospital in the gynaecology outpatient department. You also work the occasional evening shift at a family planning clinic. You live with your husband and have one grown-up daughter who lives abroad. You smoked about five cigarettes a day from when you were aged 18–22. You drink the odd gin and tonic if you go out at the weekend. You attend Zumba exercise classes every week.

Family history – There are no major health problems in your immediate family.

- Having read the information given to the simulated patient, what do you now think this station is testing?
- Make notes or discuss your thoughts with a colleague before you turn the page.

Review your approach to this station:

Tested at this station:

1. History-taking skills.
2. Communicating risk.
3. Reaching a shared management plan with an expert patient.

Domain 1 – Data gathering, technical and assessment skills

History-taking skills

This patient is asking about HRT as a means to control her perimenopausal symptoms. Before you discuss the pros and cons of treatment, you need to take a careful history to help assess whether HRT would be suitable in her case. Always remember to start with open questions and elicit the patient's ideas, concerns and expectations, before narrowing the focus of the history to specific closed questions:

- The patient thinks that she is 'going through the change'. Can she say more about this? What symptoms is she experiencing? What is happening with her periods?
- She mentions HRT. What does she know about this treatment? What are her thoughts about HRT?
- She talks about the increased risk of breast cancer, deep vein thrombosis (DVT) and PEs with HRT. Can she say more about this? What are her particular concerns?
- Does she smoke?
- Has she or any member of her immediate family ever had a DVT – 'a blood clot usually in the leg or arm' – or a PE – 'a blood clot in the lung'? Although the patient has used these acronyms, it is important to be clear exactly what you mean by them.
- Has she ever had any problems with lumps in her breasts or any abnormality on breast screening (mammography)?
- Has she ever had any gynaecological problems, such as endometriosis?
- Has she ever had any gynaecological surgery? In particular, does she still have a womb?
- Does she suffer from varicose veins or migraines?
- Does she have any other medical problems, such as diabetes or heart problems?
- How has her mood been?
- How are her symptoms affecting her work and home life?
- What was she hoping would happen from coming to the surgery today?

Domain 2 – Interpersonal skills

Communicating risk

This patient already knows that there are some added risks in taking HRT, but she is keen for you to explain these fully and hopefully reassure her that the risks are small:

- Communicating risk in terms that patients can readily understand can be a challenge to health professionals.
- Suggestions to facilitate understanding include describing absolute risk rather than relative risk, i.e. *'The risk increases from 1 in 1000 to 2 in 1000'* rather than *'The risk increases by 100%'.*
- She mentions the increased risk of breast cancer, DVTs and PEs with HRT. Does she also know about the small increased risk of stroke, ovarian cancer and endometrial cancer (the latter in those using oestrogen-only HRT)?
- The patient is concerned about her BP and previous smoking. You could reassure her that she has accumulated only one pack year of smoking, more than 25 years ago, which is unlikely to have a significant effect on the risks associated with HRT.
- Her BP has been well controlled since diagnosis, her cholesterol level is low, and she has no history of heart problems. You could advise her that although the product literature advises caution in prescribing HRT to patients with hypertension, the *British National Formulary (BNF)* states that evidence for this advice is unsatisfactory and many women with such a diagnosis may stand to benefit from HRT. However, it would be important for her to continue having her blood pressure monitored regularly. What does she think about this?
- She has specifically referred to the risks of breast cancer and thromboembolism. Would she like more detailed information on these risks?
- If so, you could go through the risk table section on HRT in the *BNF* together, explaining that about 10 in every 1000 women aged 50–59 years not using HRT have breast cancer diagnosed over 5 years, whereas in those taking combined HRT for 5 years there are about 6 extra cases per 1000 women.
- This patient had a great-aunt who developed breast cancer in her 80s. One of the cautions for use of HRT is having risk factors for oestrogen-dependent tumours, such as breast cancer in a first-degree relative. Hence only having a third-degree relative with breast cancer should not be a reason for caution. (See NICE guidelines in Further reading below for information on family history and breast cancer risk.)
- Similarly, you could go through the increased risks of thromboembolism on HRT (see Knowledge base).
- Does she understand what the figures mean in terms of small increased risks?
- Would she like written material to take away with her?
- She wants to know what you think about herbal alternatives to HRT. You could advise her that the evidence for their use is conflicting and that some can interact with prescription medications. There is also the concern regarding the quality and quantity of active ingredient in some products marketed as herbal alternatives to HRT.
- You have discussed the risks with her in some detail. Remember to advise her of the proven benefits of HRT in terms of symptomatic relief – of particular importance to her – and osteoporosis protection, together with a reduced risk of colorectal cancer (see Knowledge base).

Domain 3 – Clinical management skills

Reaching a shared management plan with an expert patient

Mrs French is an 'expert' patient in that, through her work, she already knows about indications and some of the risk factors for HRT, plus she has discussed her situation informally with a specialist medical colleague. You need to acknowledge and respond to her level of knowledge and ensure that you involve her fully in a jointly agreed management plan:

- It can sometimes feel challenging dealing with well-informed patients. Indeed, some expert patients will know more about their medical condition than their GP. The key here is not to see such patients as a threat but as an opportunity for full patient involvement in the management, including self-management, of their condition, and as a chance for health professional education, too.
- Start with general advice about lifestyle measures that may help with symptoms, such as avoiding triggers, e.g. caffeine, alcohol or certain foods, and wearing loose-fitting, cotton clothes. To slow bone loss, encourage regular weight-bearing exercise – this patient already attends dance/exercise classes twice a week.
- Having taken a thorough history and determined that there are no contraindications to the patient having HRT, and after discussing fully the risks and benefits of HRT with the patient, what are her thoughts about this treatment option?
- Explain that there are other prescribed medication alternatives to HRT (see Knowledge base) but that these are not optimal treatments and are usually considered when women cannot or do not want to take HRT.
- As she may know, options for using HRT include tablets, patches, implants, gels and vaginal rings. She has expressed an interest in patches, which you could offer to prescribe.
- Is she aware that HRT does not provide contraception and that women <50 years are considered potentially fertile for up to 2 years after their last menstrual period (and for those aged >50, for 1 year after their last menstrual period)? Is she happy with the current method of contraception she and her husband are using?
- Advise the patient that she should stop taking HRT and seek urgent medical help if she experiences any of the following:
  - sudden severe chest pain or shortness of breath
  - cough with blood-stained sputum
  - unexplained severe pain in the calf of one leg
  - serious neurological symptoms such as severe and prolonged headache, loss of vision, or weakness or numbness affecting one part of her body.
- Side effects she might experience from HRT include fluid retention, breast tenderness, headaches, breakthrough bleeding, weight gain and bloating.
- Arrange to review her in 3 months, or sooner if any problems develop.

Knowledge base – HRT

References: *BNF*, NHS Evidence Clinical Knowledge Summaries.

HRT	*Options:* • Small dose of an oestrogen • Plus a progestogen if intact uterus • Continuous combined preparations not suitable for perimenopause or within 12 months of last period (use cyclical HRT instead) • Tibolone (some androgenic action)	*Alternatives to HRT for symptomatic relief:* • Herbal remedies (conflicting evidence of effectiveness) • Clonidine (poor side-effect profile) • Antidepressants, e.g. fluoxetine, paroxetine, citalopram and venlafaxine • Gabapentin
Pros/Cons of HRT	*Pros:* • Alleviates menopausal symptoms, e.g. vaginal dryness and vasomotor instability (hot flushes, sweats) • ↓ postmenopausal osteoporosis, but should not be used solely for this purpose • ↓ risk of colorectal cancer	*Cons (small increase in risks):* • ↑ risk of breast cancer • ↑ risk of venous thromboembolism • ↑ risk of stroke • ↑ risk of ovarian cancer • ↑ risk of endometrial cancer in those using oestrogen-only HRT • ↑ risk of coronary heart disease (CHD) if started combined HRT >10 years after menopause
Management	• Treatment advised at minimum effective dose for the shortest duration • Reviewed annually • For osteoporosis, consider alternative treatments	• Should not be used to protect against cognitive function – no indication • Should not be used to prevent CHD – no indication • Experience limited with women >65 years
Risk of breast cancer	• All types of HRT ↑ risk of breast cancer within 1–2 years of starting treatment • ↑ risk related to duration of treatment • ↑ risk not related to age when starting treatment • Excess risk gone within approximately 5 years of stopping	• Baseline – about 10 in every 1000 women aged 50–59 years *not* using HRT have breast cancer diagnosed over 5 years • Combined HRT for 5 years = about 6 *extra* cases per 1000 women • Oestrogen-only HRT for 5 years = about 2 *extra* cases per 1000 women • Tibolone ↑ risk of breast cancer, but to lesser extent than combined HRT
Risk of DVT/PE	• Combined or oestrogen-only HRT ↑ risk of DVT and PE especially in first year of treatment • If predisposing factors present – personal or family history of DVT/PE, severe varicose veins, obesity, trauma or prolonged bed-rest – review need for HRT as risks may outweigh benefits	• Baseline – about 5 in every 1000 women aged 50–59 years *not* using HRT develop venous thromboembolism over 5 years • Combined HRT for 5 years = about 7 *extra* cases per 1000 women • Oestrogen-only HRT for 5 years = about 2 *extra* cases per 1000 women

(continued)

continued

Cautions and contra-indications	*Contra-indications include:*	*Cautions include:*
	• oestrogen-dependent cancer • history of breast cancer • active thrombophlebitis • recent or active angina or myocardial infarction • DVT or recurrent thromboembolism (unless anticoagulated) • liver disease • undiagnosed vaginal bleeding	• prolonged exposure to unopposed oestrogen may ↑ risk of endometrial cancer • history of breast nodules or fibrocystic disease • breast cancer in first-degree relative • factors ↑ risk of thromboembolism • migraine • diabetes (increased risk of heart disease)

Take-home messages

- For the treatment of menopausal symptoms the benefits of short-term HRT outweigh the risks for the majority of women.
- Explaining risks to patients in terms they can understand is a skill that can be readily assessed in the Clinical Skills Assessment (CSA).
- A consultation with an expert patient should be seen as an opportunity for full patient participation.

Tasks

- Re-run the scenario with the patient having two sisters with breast cancer diagnosed at a young age.
- Re-run the scenario with the patient complaining of post-coital bleeding.
- Re-run the scenario with the patient aged 38 with FSH and LH raised (i.e. suspected early menopause).
- Re-run the scenario with the patient presenting with hot flushes and vaginal dryness aged 56, with her last period 5 years previously.

1-minute explanations for patients

- Explain how HRT works.
- Explain why patients without a uterus (e.g. post-hysterectomy) can have a different type of HRT.
- Explain why some HRT preparations are 'cyclical'.

Ideas for further revision

Make sure you are able to explain the risks and benefits associated with a range of interventions in primary care, such as prescribing combined and progestogen-only hormonal contraceptives, HRT, aspirin, and steroid use, together with the pros and cons of undertaking certain tests, such as a prostate-specific antigen (PSA) test.

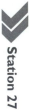

Further reading

British Menopause Society Council Consensus Statement on Hormone Replacement Therapy 2008 www.thebms.org.uk/statementpreview.php?id=1

British National Formulary (BNF). Published jointly by BMJ Publishing Group and RPS Publishing, London. Updated every 6 months www.bnf.org

Menopause Matters – an independent, clinician-led website www.menopausematters.co.uk

NHS Evidence Clinical Knowledge Summaries – Menopause management www.cks.nhs.uk

NICE quick reference guide on familial breast cancer (Guideline 41) 2006 www.nice.org.uk/nicemedia/pdf/CG41quickrefguide1.pdf

RCGP curriculum statement 10.1 – Women's health www.rcgp.org.uk

STATION 28

Information given to candidates

Barry Southgate is a 20-year-old who has recently registered at your practice.

Last week he saw the practice nurse for a new patient check and told her that he has been taking heroin for 18 months, but now wants to 'kick the habit'.

The nurse noted:

Smoker	10 roll-up cigarettes a day
Alcohol	Rarely
Height	170 cm
Weight	51 kg
Body mass index (BMI)	17.6 kg/m²
Urinalysis	Normal
Blood pressure (BP)	126/72 mmHg

Your practice has a shared care arrangement with the local specialist addiction unit. One of your GP colleagues, Dr Black, together with support from the local drugs service, runs a weekly clinic in the GP surgery, in which opiate replacement treatment is routinely prescribed.

As the patient walks into the consultation room he says, 'I really want to get off the heroin, and need your help, doc.'

- What do you think this station is testing?
- Make notes or discuss your thoughts with a colleague before you read on.

Plan your approach to this station:

Information given to simulated patient

Basic details – You are Barry Southgate, a 20-year-old former labourer.

Appearance and behaviour – You are a little agitated and fidgety during the consultation. You are underweight. You make good eye contact and are casually dressed in clothes that are overdue for a change.

History

Freely divulged to doctor – You have been using heroin continuously for about 18 months, at first smoking and then injecting. You have never sought help for this before. You thought you were in control of things, but having lost your job and split up with your partner because of your drug use, you realize that you need help. You are hoping that the doctor can prescribe you some methadone today.

Divulged to doctor if specifically asked – To begin with you were funding your drug use from your wages and by borrowing money, but since you lost your job 1 year ago you have been shoplifting as a source of money to buy drugs. You have been cautioned by the police, but have never been to prison. You have not been to hospital as the result of an overdose or any other drug-related problem. Over the last 4 months you have started occasionally injecting into your groin, as you find it increasingly difficult to find veins elsewhere in your arms or legs. You have shared needles with your brother on several occasions. You have not been tested or vaccinated for hepatitis or HIV.

Ideas, concerns and expectations – Two weeks ago one of your friends had an overdose when injecting heroin after being released from prison. You were with him when this happened. You called 999 but were scared that the police might be involved, so you did not stay for the ambulance. You have heard that he is ok, but this incident has made you think about your own drug use – you are worried that the same thing could happen to you and want to get help to tackle your problem. Initially you will be annoyed if the doctor says you cannot start methadone today. However, if the doctor explains why this is the case, and is understanding of your circumstances, you will agree to come to the dedicated clinic at the surgery. You will be happy to accept any offers of testing for HIV or hepatitis, and hepatitis vaccinations, which you have been meaning to have done for some time. You do not want to think about seeking help from housing or welfare projects yet, until you are more stable on methadone and off heroin.

First words spoken to doctor – 'I really want to get off the heroin, and need your help, doc.'

Medical history – You have never had any problems with infected injection sites or abscesses. You have not had any blood clots in your limbs or lungs. You have lost nearly 3 stones in weight over the last year as you often go without meals. Your teeth have been giving you trouble lately, but the heroin helps with the pain. You were fit and well before you started taking heroin.

Drug history – You are currently using two to three £10 bags of heroin a day, injecting three times a day. About twice a week you smoke crack cocaine and you use cannabis to help 'come down' from the crack. Before you tried heroin you used to take speed (amphetamines) and ecstasy. As far as you know you are not allergic to any medication.

Social history – You split up with your partner 6 months ago, after repeatedly arguing about your drug use, and have been staying with various friends since then. You do not have any children. You have spent the odd night sleeping on the streets when you could not find accommodation. Your mother has said she won't speak to you again until you are drug-free as you started to steal from her to fund your heroin use. You smoke about 10 roll-up cigarettes a day. You hardly ever drink alcohol. You have not worked for the last year, ever since your heroin use got out of control and you were sacked for being off sick regularly. You do not drive.

Family history – Your father died of alcohol-related liver problems in his 50s. You have one brother who is currently in prison for burglary. He has had a blood clot in his leg through injecting into his groin.

- Having read the information given to the simulated patient, what do you now think this station is testing?
- Make notes or discuss your thoughts with a colleague before you turn the page.

Review your approach to this station:

Tested at this station:

1. Ability to engage constructively with a patient who misuses drugs.
2. Taking a drug misuse history.
3. Physical examination.
4. Recognizing limits of competence.
5. Management of first presentation of drug misuse.

Domain 1 – Interpersonal skills

Ability to engage constructively with a patient who misuses drugs

The most important goal with patients who misuse drugs is to try to engender a sense of trust and hope, so that they will engage with services and return to see you for follow-up care:

- Be empathetic and find out about the patient's agenda. What are his ideas, concerns and expectations from coming to see you today?
- Drug-using patients have the right to access good quality services. You must demonstrate a non-judgemental approach and not let any personal opinion of a perceived self-inflicted problem affect his care.
- Encourage hope – positively affirm his actions in taking the important first steps to address his drug use by coming down to the surgery today.
- Explain that change is not easy and that he may have relapses along the way, but the important thing is that he is motivated and wants to change.
- Explain that prescribing methadone – or any equivalent opiate replacement medication – is only one part of a package of care that needs to be put in place to help support him, once a full assessment has been done.

Domain 2 – Data gathering, technical and assessment skills

Taking a drug misuse history

You need to tailor your history to cover the pertinent issues surrounding the patient's drug misuse:

- Start with open questions. Can he tell you more about his drug use? What impact has it had on his life?
- More specific questions which may help give a detailed picture of the patient's drug use include:
  1. Drugs:
     - What drugs does he use? How much of each does he use? How long has he been using each one?
     - Remember also specifically to ask about cannabis and alcohol use, as these are often not seen as relevant by patients who misuse drugs.
     - Does he inject or smoke each drug? If he injects, does he ever share needles or injecting equipment? Where does he inject?

- How much does he use of each drug each day, or per week? Where does he get the drugs from?
- Does he take the drugs on his own or with others?

2. Treatment:
   - Any previous treatment for his drug use?
   - Has he had any periods of being drug-free since he started?

3. Physical and mental problems:
   - Any physical problems as a result of his drug use, such as clots, abscesses or infections? Has he ever had a drug overdose?
   - Does he suffer from asthma? Inhaled drugs and stimulants can exacerbate asthma.
   - Any time in hospital as a result of his drug use?
   - Any mental health problems, such as depression or self-harm? Has he ever seen a mental health specialist such as a psychiatrist?

4. Forensic history:
   - Has he ever been involved with the criminal justice system as a result of his drug use? For example, time in prison or on a community drugs order, or on probation?
   - Are there any court cases pending? Being engaged with drugs services may help with sentencing and could be a reason for presenting now.

5. Vaccinations and testing:
   - Has he had any blood tests for viruses such as hepatitis or HIV?
   - Has he been vaccinated for hepatitis? Can he remember which type – A or B? What about tetanus vaccination?

6. Social situation:
   - Where is he living at the moment? Has he ever been homeless as a result of his drug use?
   - Does he have a partner? Are there any children living with him or visiting regularly?
   - Is he working?

- Remember, the list above is only a guide. It is more important that you respond to the patient's agenda and concerns, and demonstrate an empathetic and understanding approach, rather than simply ask a checklist of questions.

Physical examination

When a drug user first presents it is good practice to examine him for evidence of drug use, e.g. needle track marks, and also to make sure that he has no problems such as abscesses or a deep vein thrombosis. Are there any signs of intoxication today? You should also assess his mental state. Is the patient depressed? Does he represent a suicide risk? At this station you will not have to actually physically examine the patient. However, you would be expected to attempt to examine him, at which point the examiner will tell you the findings – namely, that there are needle track marks on the patient's arms and that he is thin, but that otherwise examination is normal.

Domain 3 – Clinical management skills

Recognizing limits of competence

The Department of Health guidelines (see Further reading below) make clear that all doctors should be equipped to deal with drug-related issues. However, for the GP inexperienced in dealing with patients who misuse drugs, this might mean appropriate support, advice and general medical care, plus referral to a GP colleague or the local specialist drugs service for further management:

- Acknowledge his desire to start medication straight away, but explain that your practice works in partnership with the local specialist drugs service in offering a dedicated clinic once a week, here at the surgery, at which your colleague, Dr Black, can prescribe heroin replacement treatment, such as methadone or buprenorphine, if this is appropriate. Do not feel pressurized by the patient into prescribing outside the limits of your competence.
- Explain that there is still much that you can help with today, and that at the end of the consultation you could help book an appointment for him at Dr Black's next clinic.
- It is far better in the first consultation with a drug user to show empathy and support, and make clear that the patient's needs will be addressed, than be rushed into prescribing before a full and proper assessment has been undertaken.

Management of first presentation of drug misuse

There is much that you can offer a patient who first presents with problem drug use. But remember that you have only 10 minutes for the station, so you need to be focused:

- Despite not being in a position to prescribe opioid replacement treatment to the patient today, you should still do the following:
  - Offer basic harm-minimization advice and health promotion, e.g.
    - safer injecting advice – not to share; use clean needles; avoid the groin or neck; not to inject on own
    - needle exchange information
    - sexual health advice, e.g. encourage condom use
    - screening for blood-borne viruses (hepatitis B, C and HIV).
  - Offer hepatitis A and B, plus tetanus vaccination. The RCGP recommends opportunistic vaccination rather than waiting to check serology first.
  - Offer general medical care, e.g. smoking cessation advice, dietary advice.
  - Signpost him to other services, for example:
    - Citizen's Advice Bureau for benefits advice
    - local authority or homelessness project for housing advice
    - local National Health Service (NHS) dentist for an assessment.
- You could explain that before opioid replacement treatment, such as methadone or buprenorphine, is prescribed, it is usual for a urine sample to be taken to confirm opiate use. You could offer to take a sample now and send it off for toxicology, as this might help speed things up when he attends Dr Black's clinic.
- Doctors are expected to report cases where they are providing structured drug treatment for substance dependence to their local National Drug Treatment Monitoring System. This should probably occur when the patient starts on

treatment (if appropriate) from your colleague Dr Black. For more details see the *British National Formulary (BNF)* section in Further reading.

Knowledge base

Reference: GP curriculum statement 15.3, citing *Task Force to Review Services for Drug Misusers* – see Further reading below for details.

Hierarchy of goals of drug treatment

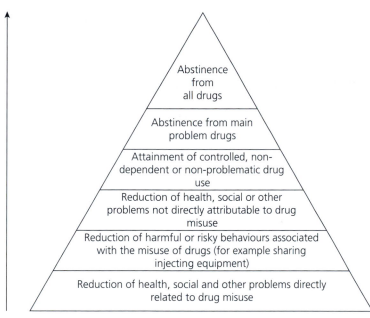

Abstinence from all drugs

Abstinence from main problem drugs

Attainment of controlled, non-dependent or non-problematic drug use

Reduction of health, social or other problems not directly attributable to drug misuse

Reduction of harmful or risky behaviours associated with the misuse of drugs (for example sharing injecting equipment)

Reduction of health, social and other problems directly related to drug misuse

---

Take-home messages

- Drug-using patients have complex problems and you should try to address their social, psychological and physical needs.
- You should prescribe for drug misuse only within the limits of your competence and refer to GP colleagues with appropriate training or specialist centres for further management.
- There is still much that you can do to help drug-using patients presenting in primary care.

Tasks

- Re-run the scenario with the patient reporting that he is already being prescribed 90 mg methadone OD from his local drugs service (in another city) but that he is staying for a few days with his sister and has lost his medication.
- Re-run the scenario with the patient returning from an overseas trip to Thailand where he reports having smoked heroin.
- Re-run the scenario with the patient's mother attending on her own, to discuss her concerns about her son's drug use. Think about how you might offer support to her.

1-minute explanations for patients

- Explain how methadone works.
- Explain why sharing equipment other than needles (e.g. spoons) can still carry risks.
- Explain the treatment for hepatitis C.

Ideas for further revision

The GP curriculum statement on drug and alcohol problems suggests that GP specialty registrars should be encouraged to look after some of their practice's drug-using patients and follow them through their patient journey. In addition, you may find the interactive RCGP e-learning modules on substance misuse helpful (see Further reading).

Further reading

British Medical Association and Royal Pharmaceutical Society of Great Britain. *The British National Formulary 63* Section: Guidance of prescribing – Controlled drugs and drug dependence; notification of patients receiving structured drug treatment for substance dependence. London: BMJ Books, March 2012 www.bnf.org/bnf/index.htm

Department of Health (England), the Scottish Government, Welsh Assembly Government and Northern Ireland Executive. *Drug Misuse and Dependence: UK Guidelines on Clinical Management* London: The Stationery Office, 2007 (so-called 'Orange Book')

Latest government policy, legislation and guidance on alcohol and drug use www.homeoffice.gov.uk/drugs/

National Institute of Health and Clinical Excellence. *Drug misuse: opioid detoxification*. London: NICE, 2007 http://publications.nice.org.uk/drug-misuse-cg52

NHS National Library for Health Clinical Knowledge Summaries – Opioid dependence www.cks.nhs.uk/opioid_dependence

RCGP curriculum statement 15.3 – Clinical management: drug and alcohol problems www.rcgp.org.uk

RCGP substance misuse interactive e-learning modules: Harm Reduction; and, Treatment Planning (form part of RCGP Certificate in the Management of Drug Misuse part 1) www.elearning.rcgp.org.uk

Rushforth B, Wright N. New approaches to dealing with opioid dependence. *BJGP* 2011; 61: 710–711

Substance Misuse Management in General Practice www.smmgp.org.uk

Task Force to Review Services for Drug Misusers: report of an Independent Survey of Drug Treatment Services in England. London: Department of Health, 1996

Information given to candidates

Johan Slemick is a 72-year-old retired insurance broker.

He saw your GP colleague, Dr Umesh, 10 days ago with a history of haemoptysis, worsening cough and weight loss.

He has smoked 20 cigarettes a day for 50 years.

The patient's notes state that he has chronic obstructive pulmonary disease (COPD) and is prescribed:

- salbutamol metered dose inhaler (MDI) 100 µg – 2 puffs BD
- tiotropium 18 µg (one dry powder inhalation) OD
- salmeterol MDI 25 µg – 2 puffs BD

Examination 10 days ago revealed reduced air entry at the right lung base.

Dr Umesh requested an urgent chest x-ray and asked the patient to return to discuss the findings.

The chest x-ray report reads:

'There is a large (3 cm diameter) suspicious-looking shadow in the right hilar area. The lungs are hyper-expanded, consistent with a diagnosis of COPD. Given the patient's smoking history and current symptoms, there is a high probability of neoplastic pathology. Suggest referral for urgent computed tomography (CT).

Dr Umesh is on holiday this week so the patient has been booked in with you.

As the patient enters the room he says, 'Hello, doctor, I got a call asking me to come in to discuss my chest x-ray result.'

- What do you think this station is testing?
- Make notes or discuss your thoughts with a colleague before you read on.

Plan your approach to this station:

Information given to simulated patient

Basic details – You are Johan Slemick, a 72-year-old retired insurance broker.

Appearance and behaviour – At first you appear relaxed and confident. However, when the doctor tells you the chest x-ray result, you are initially distressed (despite having suspected that it might be something serious – see Ideas, concerns and expectations below).

History

Freely divulged to doctor – You had been meaning to come to the doctor's for some time as your cough has been getting worse over the last 2–3 months. Then, 10 days ago, you coughed up bright fresh blood. You have never coughed up blood before, so you came straight down to the surgery. The doctor examined you and arranged for a chest x-ray. Yesterday you had one more episode of coughing up blood. As before, this was a small to medium amount of bright red blood.

Divulged to doctor if specifically asked – You have lost about one and a half stones in weight over the last few months, but as you were overweight to begin with you thought this could only be a good thing. Your appetite has been poor for the last month. You always suffered from a 'smoker's cough' and see the doctor for antibiotics for 'bronchitis' at least a couple of times a year. You have not had any chest infections recently, although you do feel a bit more 'out of puff'. You have not had any chest pain. If the doctor says that the x-ray suggests that things could be serious, you will ask directly whether it is cancer. Despite usually being the sort of person who wants to know all about your health, today you will initially say – when told that it could be cancer – that you don't want to know any more details. But if the doctor appears kind and understanding, and asks more about your concerns, you will disclose your worries at this news and agree to come back and see the doctor in a few days to discuss your options. You do not want to talk today about any more tests as you just want to 'get your head' round the possibility that it could be very serious. You do not want your wife told at this stage.

Ideas, concerns and expectations – When you coughed up blood you started to feel uneasy about what was going on. You were hoping that it was due to the 'bronchitis'. Neither yourself nor the doctor you saw last time mentioned that it might be something serious, but it worried you that he marked the x-ray card 'Urgent'. It was then that you thought it might be cancer. An old work friend died from lung cancer a couple of years ago, and you remember that it had started with him coughing up blood. You have been trying to tell yourself that it's going to be ok, but deep down you feel less confident. All sorts of negative thoughts have been going through your mind, such as how your wife would cope if you became ill, and whether you will be well enough to go on the cruise you have booked for both of you in 4 months' time. You have been praying that the doctor would say today that the chest x-ray was fine and that it could all be put down to the 'bronchitis'.

First words spoken to doctor – 'Hello, doctor, I got a call asking me to come in to discuss my chest x-ray result.'

Medical history – For about 10 years you have been using inhalers to help with the damage done to your lungs through smoking. Otherwise you have been fairly healthy and have never had any serious illnesses.

Drug history – You have been using a blue inhaler (salbutamol), one or two puffs a couple of times a day, for about 10 years. A second inhaler, tiotropium, one inhalation once a day, was added 2 years ago, and last year your doctor also started you on a salmeterol inhaler – two puffs twice a day – to help with your worsening breathlessness. You are not allergic to any medication.

Social history – You have smoked since your early 20s – about 20 cigarettes a day. You have never seriously considered giving up smoking, as you 'really enjoy it'. You drink the occasional glass of wine with meals. You live with your wife, who has been suffering with her own health and mobility problems recently – last year she lost the sight in one eye due to a stroke and also fell and broke her hip. You were both looking forward to a month's cruise in the Caribbean in 4 months' time. You have a grown-up son who lives in Spain.

Family history – There are no major health problems in your immediate family

- Having read the information given to the simulated patient, what do you now think this station is testing?
- Make notes or discuss your thoughts with a colleague before you turn the page.

Review your approach to this station:

Tested at this station:

1. Breaking bad news.
2. Negotiating with a patient regarding further management.

Domains 1 and 2 – Interpersonal skills and data gathering

Breaking bad news

Although there is no definite diagnosis at this stage, the chest x-ray result, together with the patient's history, is highly suspicious of a sinister pathology. You need to use skill and tact when breaking this bad news to the patient:

- Ask the patient to explain what first brought him to the surgery.
- Clarify events since he last saw your colleague.
- Explore his understanding of why the x-ray was requested.
- From his answers to the above it should become clear whether the patient suspects a worrying finding. If not, then a more direct question would be useful, such as: *'Have you thought about what the problem might be?'*
- Explore whether he is the type of person who likes to know all about his medical test results. Be careful not to impose information on a patient who gives verbal or non-verbal cues that he is reluctant to be told more.
- If the patient does appear to suspect something serious, you need to explore in more detail his understanding about what the diagnosis could be.
- But if the patient appears not to have considered a serious pathology, then firing a warning shot will help in the process of breaking the bad news, e.g. *'I'm afraid the chest x-ray result is somewhat worrying'.*
- You may not have a firm diagnosis yet, but it is still important to explain the chest x-ray result fully and honestly, but without extinguishing hope.
- Give information in manageable chunks. Use pauses between chunks to allow the patient time to process his thoughts.
- Use silences to give the patient space to go at his own pace.
- Once you have disclosed the information about the chest x-ray findings, it is important to acknowledge and thereby give permission for any distress, e.g. *'I can see that you are very distressed at this news'.*
- Ask about the patient's concerns and feelings at the news.
- If he asks you directly whether it is cancer, do not side-step the question but explain that further tests would need to be done but that lung cancer is a strong possibility.
- Again ask whether he has any further concerns. Do not move on to management options with a patient until you have elicited all the patient's concerns. In this case, he is particularly worried about what will happen to his wife if he becomes ill and whether he will be well enough to go on the upcoming cruise.
- Acknowledge that at this stage the diagnosis and prognosis are uncertain, and empathize at the distress this uncertainty itself may cause.

Domain 3 – Clinical management skills
Negotiating with a patient regarding further management

After breaking bad news and fully addressing the patient's concerns it is important to negotiate about how to proceed:

- Emphasize the fact that although the chest x-ray result is worrying, you will not have a firm diagnosis until further investigations are done.
- This patient does not want to discuss further tests today. Make sure you respect this and do not force information on him about CT scans or referral to hospital.
- Explore why he feels this way and ask whether he would like to come back to see you in a few days to discuss things further.
- Although you need to respect his wishes not to discuss things further today, it is important to stress the importance of him seeing you again very soon. You could offer to book an appointment for a couple of days' time while he is with you today.
- Many patients, once they have heard that the diagnosis could be cancer, do not fully take in information about further tests or treatment options. So as well as respecting his views, it may be useful to go over these at another appointment.
- Would he like to bring someone with him to the next appointment to provide support?
- You could also offer either to tell his wife or to be present when he tells her if he decides at some future point to discuss it with her.
- He may find it helpful to keep a note of any questions that come to him before seeing you again.
- How is he going to get home today? Is there anyone who could come to pick him up?

Knowledge base

From Faulkner, A. ABC of palliative care: Communication with patients, families, and other professionals. *BMJ* 1998; 316: 130–132. Reproduced with permission from BMJ Publishing Group.

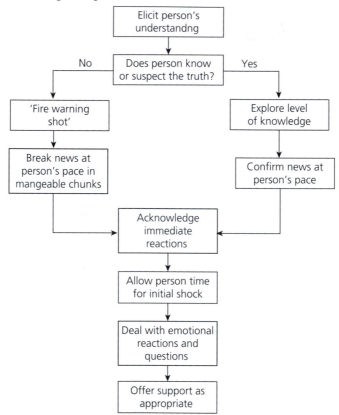

Recommended manner of breaking bad news

Take-home messages

- Never force information on patients unless they indicate that they want to know more.
- Breaking bad news can be emotionally draining for the doctor, too. Debriefing with colleagues can help manage negative feelings generated by such consultations.

Tasks

- Re-run the scenario with the patient in denial that there is likely to be anything seriously wrong and he keeps saying that the x-ray findings are probably due to his 'bronchitis'.
- Re-run the scenario with the patient in tears and distressed by the news. Think how you would manage this emotionally charged consultation.
- Re-run the scenario with the patient consulting on his own and not having very good English. What further challenges might this bring?

1-minute explanations for patients

- Explain what a CT scan involves.
- Explain what bronchoscopy involves.
- Explain the wording of the chest x-ray report (i.e. go through it with someone role-playing the patient).

Ideas for further revision

Hospital posts that form part of GP specialty training programmes, such as emergency medicine and elderly care, regularly require doctors to break bad news. You could first ask to sit in with an experienced, senior colleague. Then ask whether they will sit in with you while you take the lead, and provide feedback on the consultation. Additionally, you could simulate such scenarios with peers or your trainer, or request formal sessions with fellow GP trainees using trained actors to take the patients' roles.

Further reading

Dunphy J. *Communication in Palliative Care*. Oxford: Radcliffe, 2011

Faulkner A. ABC of palliative care: Communication with patients, families, and other professionals. *BMJ* 1998; 316: 130–132 www.bmj.com

Maguire, P. *Communication Skills for Doctors*. London: Arnold, 2000. Chapter 6: Breaking bad news

NICE. Chronic obstructive pulmonary disease (update): quick reference guide, 2010 www.nice.org.uk/guidance/CG101/QuickRefGuide

RCGP curriculum statement 12 – care of people with cancer & palliative care www.rcgp.org.uk

Information given to candidates

Candidates note: this station is a **home visit**. In the exam you will be escorted by an invigilator to a room made to look like a patient's living room. The consultation will take place there.

> Ibrahim Abboud is a 42-year-old male patient who has recently registered with your practice.
>
> There is no medical history available and the receptionist has recorded the following information:
>
> *Home visit requested for Ibrahim Abboud – new patient. Never been registered with a GP in UK before. Friend has requested home visit as patient unable to leave home. No telephone details available.*

As you enter the room you are greeted by the patient: 'Thank you for coming to see me, doctor. My friend said he would ask you to visit.'

- What do you think this station is testing?
- Make notes or discuss your thoughts with a colleague before you read on.

Plan your approach to this station:

Information given to simulated patient

Basic details – You are Ibrahim Abboud, a 42-year-old Black African. You have been living in the UK for 6 weeks and are seeking political asylum. You are living with a friend who delivered your practice registration to the surgery and arranged for a GP to come and assess you at home as you are unable to go out alone.

Appearance and behaviour – You are withdrawn and quietly spoken. Your tone and body language show you are anxious, particularly when asked to divulge details about your life in Africa and how you came to be in the UK. You are initially cautious when asked to answer questions and do so with little animation. If you feel rushed and pressured you will become increasingly anxious and provide only short, factual responses, but if the doctor makes you feel at ease then you will divulge more about your circumstances and feelings.

History

Freely divulged to doctor – You need help because every time you leave the house alone you feel very unwell. You feel short of breath and your heart begins to race. You also feel dizzy to the extent that you need to find something to lean against. This happens every time you try to leave the house unless your friend is with you.

Divulged to doctor if specifically asked – The symptoms first occurred during the journey to the UK. You came to the UK by boat, having fled your home nation after you were arrested by the police for your political views. You do not want to talk about what happened in prison. On arrival you applied for asylum and the process is ongoing. You have support from a case worker, who you see every week, and she advised you to register with a GP. The worst episode occurred 3 weeks ago after you were moved to your current residence, when you attempted to travel by bus. Several young people at the bus stop started to laugh at you when you asked which bus to take into town and this escalated to them pushing you and taking your money. Since this incident you have managed to go out of the house alone on only one occasion. When you did you immediately felt dizzy and developed tightness in your chest. You were taking fast, shallow breaths and began to feel faint and sick. The symptoms resolved when you got back to the house. Even the thought of trying to leave the house now makes you feel dizzy and your heart rate increases. You are finding it difficult to sleep at night, with recurrent nightmares about what happened when you were in prison. During the day you can have flashbacks to when you were arrested. You have had no thoughts of self-harm.

Ideas, concerns and expectations – You are scared about what is happening and are initially wary about trusting the doctor. You think your symptoms are a physical manifestation of what happened in prison and wonder whether your heart has been damaged beyond repair. You struggle to understand the concepts of stress and anxiety as you believe consciousness resides in the heart and not the mind. If the doctor can give you some medication to help, you will be grateful. Talking to someone about what has happened fills you with fear, but you may be willing to be referred for this if the doctor explains how this might help you.

First words spoken to doctor – 'Thank you for coming to see me, doctor. My friend said he would ask you to visit.'

Medical history – You have no other significant medical history.

Drug history – You do not take any regular medication.

Social history – You are married with three children. Your wife and children live in your ancestral village away from danger. You have had no contact with them since you left your country. You had been living in the capital city working as a journalist when you were arrested. You do not smoke or drink alcohol. Currently you are living with a friend who was granted asylum last year. He also finds it difficult to talk openly about the situation in your home country.

Family history – There are no major illnesses in your immediate family.

- Having read the information given to the simulated patient, what do you now think this station is testing?
- Make notes or discuss your thoughts with a colleague before you turn the page.

Review your approach to this station:

Tested at this station:

1. Dealing with sensitive issues.
2. Understanding a patient's illness experience.
3. Taking a psychiatric history.
4. Negotiating a shared management plan.

Domain 1 – Interpersonal skills

Dealing with sensitive issues

This station is highly dependent on a candidate's ability to build trust by allowing time and space for the patient to divulge their story. Awareness that significant cultural differences may exist in the doctor–patient relationship is also important and particular care needs to be taken over how the patient's ideas, concerns and expectations are elicited.

- The use of open questions is vital in this situation in order to facilitate a patient-centred consultation.
- It may be necessary to ask more than one open question on the same topic to encourage the patient to divulge their story.
- Non-verbal communication and the use of silence are necessary techniques to encourage the patient to be as open as they feel comfortable.
- Signposting closed questions and explaining the purpose for probing deeper into any relevant issue can help reduce a sense of interrogation. Repeatedly asking 'How did that make you feel?' when trying to understand the patient's experience is also likely to feel interrogative.
- Acknowledging the patient's distress and emphasizing that you are there to help can build trust.
- There is a strong likelihood that this patient is a victim of torture. In situations such as this it is important to exercise caution regarding physical proximity and touch. Specific consent and thorough explanation are advisable for any physical examination.
- The clinical environment can also be a stressor for victims of torture as medical instruments and clinical rooms can appear similar to those used for torture.

Domain 2 – Data gathering, technical and assessment skills

Understanding a patient's illness experience

In cross-cultural consultations it is important to check you have correctly understood what a patient has said. Health and illness beliefs can vary considerably, even within one's own culture, and it is therefore necessary to avoid making assumptions.

When traumatic and distressing events have occurred it is possible that a patient is unwilling to discuss them at length during an initial clinical encounter. Building trust is more important for understanding a patient's experience than trying to gather all the information within a single consultation.

Taking a psychiatric history

Physical and psychological trauma can manifest in many different ways, such as depression, generalized anxiety disorder, substance misuse, post-traumatic stress disorder (PTSD) and medically unexplained symptoms. Differentiating between these is dependent on being able to elicit sufficient relevant information about signs and symptoms:

- The duration and persistence of symptoms along with an accurate chronological account of their development is important.
- Poor sleep pattern is widely recognized as a symptom of depression, but identifying that this is related to recurrent nightmares provides a clue for a possible diagnosis of PTSD.
- Pre occupation with specific thoughts can be suggestive of anxiety or again a sign of PTSD if vivid flashbacks are occurring.
- Assess the risk of self-harm and suicide in all patients presenting with psychological distress.
- Identify the severity of symptoms both as perceived by the patient and by exploration of their functional impact.

Domain 3 – Clinical management skills

Negotiating a shared management plan

The signs and symptoms in the scenario are suggestive of a diagnosis of PTSD. Before a management plan can be agreed it is helpful to provide a culturally relevant explanation of the possible diagnosis.

- PTSD is a relatively common and under-recognized response to frightening or distressing situations.
- Persistent reliving of a stressor, avoidance or emotional numbing and hyperarousal symptoms feature in the diagnostic criteria.
- Symptoms often develop immediately after a distressing event but can be delayed until much later.
- Treatment options include watchful waiting, pharmacotherapy and psychological therapies. Does the patient have any preferences on how to proceed?
- In some people PTSD can resolve without treatment. This is more likely if the incident related to onset occurred less than 6 weeks ago, symptoms are mild and improving at the time of consultation.
- The National Institute for Health and Clinical Excellence (NICE) guidance on PTSD strongly recommends that drug treatments should not be used first-line in preference to trauma-focused psychological therapy but can be useful if delays in accessing psychological treatments are likely.
- Antidepressant drugs (paroxetine or mirtazapine) are licensed for PTSD and should be considered when a patient chooses not to engage in psychological therapy.
- Does the patient want more time to consider the options outlined today?

Knowledge base – The diagnosis of PTSD

Screening questionnaires for PTSD, such as the Trauma Screening Questionnaire can be employed to help aid diagnosis. From Brewin, CR *et al.* Brief screening instrument for post traumatic stress disorder. *British Journal of Psychiatry* 2002; 181: 158–162. Reproduced with permission.

Instructions: Please consider the following reactions which sometimes occur after a traumatic event. This questionnaire is concerned with your personal reactions to the traumatic event which happened to you. Please indicate (Yes/No) whether or not you have experienced any of the following at least twice in the past week:		
	Yes	No
1. Upsetting thoughts or memories about the event that have come into your mind against your will.		
2. Upsetting dreams about the event.		
3. Acting or feeling as though the event were happening again.		
4. Feeling upset by reminders of the event.		
5. Bodily reactions (such as fast heartbeat, stomach churning, sweatiness, dizziness) when reminded of the event.		
6. Difficulty falling or staying asleep.		
7. Irritability or outbursts of anger.		
8. Difficulty concentrating.		
9. Heightened awareness of potential dangers to yourself and others.		
10. Being jumpy or being startled at something unexpected.		

If the person has six or more positive responses, they are at risk of having PTSD and further assessment should be undertaken. There are numerous structured interview tools available and the decision on which to use is often governed by the referral routes available.

Access to National Health Services (NHS) for asylum seekers

Guidance exists from the Department of Health outlining who is entitled to free NHS services in England. The British Medical Association (BMA) has provided further clarification of the various entitlements and means of accessing healthcare for asylum seekers and refused asylum seekers in the UK (see Further reading). The key points from this clarification are reproduced below:

- All asylum seekers and refugees are entitled to register with a GP and to receive free NHS hospital treatment.
- GP practices retain the discretion to register refused asylum seekers to the same extent that they have this discretion in relation to registering any patient, regardless of his or her residency status.
- Treatment of certain specified communicable diseases (e.g. TB, hepatitis B and measles), compulsory mental health treatment and treatment provided in an emergency department are exempt from charges for all patients.
- Health professionals must not discriminate against asylum seekers or refuse asylum seekers by unfairly prioritizing other patients in preference to them.

- In England, refused asylum seekers and asylum seekers who are not receiving benefits may still be entitled to free prescriptions.
- Different entitlements to free hospital treatment for refused asylum seekers exist in each of the UK nations.
- It is not the responsibility of doctors to make decisions on the eligibility of patients for free NHS hospital care.
- Refused asylum seekers who were undergoing a course of hospital treatment at the time their claim for asylum was rejected are entitled to receive that period of treatment free of charge until completion.
- Asylum seekers and refused asylum seekers have the same rights to medical confidentiality as other patients.

The following definitions may be helpful when seeking to understand the various stages of the asylum process (see www.refugeecouncil.org.uk for further details):

Refugee: A person who, owing to well-founded fear of being persecuted for reasons of race, religion, nationality, membership of a particular social group or political opinion, is outside the country of his nationality and is unable or, owing to such fear, unwilling to avail himself of the protection of that country; or who, not having a nationality and being outside the country of his former habitual residence as a result of such events, is unable or, owing to such fear, unwilling to return to it. (*The 1951 United Nations Convention Relating to the Status of Refugees*)

Asylum seeker: A person who has left his or her country of origin and formally applied for asylum in another country but whose application has not yet been concluded.

Refused asylum seeker: A person whose asylum application has been unsuccessful and who has no other claim for protection awaiting a decision. Some refused asylum seekers voluntarily return home, others are forcibly returned, and for some it is not safe or practical for them to return until conditions in their country change.

'Illegal' immigrant: Someone whose entry into or presence in a country contravenes immigration laws.

Take-home messages

- PTSD can be difficult to diagnose and only a minority of cases respond to watchful waiting.
- Cross-cultural consultations have many challenges and care must be taken to ensure all parties understand what is being said.
- Asylum seekers and refugees often have difficulties accessing healthcare.

Tasks

- Re-run the scenario as a station requiring an interpreter. Finding two colleagues who are fluent in a language can make this very realistic.
- Re-run the scenario with the patient presenting with symptoms of depression.

- Re-run the scenario with the patient expressing concern about the safety of their family in the country of origin.
- Re-run the scenario with the patient presenting with symptoms suggestive of stable angina. What further issues regarding referral pathways might this raise?

1-minute explanations for patients

- Describe a diagnosis of panic disorder.
- Describe the difference between psychology and psychiatry.
- Explain how and why antidepressant therapy should be gradually reduced if withdrawal is planned.

Ideas for further revision

Developing insight into the different cultural perspectives of mental health problems is important. Take some time to discuss this with peers from different ethnic origins and compare your findings with some of the web-based information.

Further reading

Brewin, CR *et al*. Brief screening instrument for post traumatic stress disorder. *British Journal of Psychiatry* 2002; 181: 158–162

British Medical Association. *Access to Health Care For Asylum Seekers and Refused Asylum Seekers – Guidance for Doctors*. London, 2012

National Collaborating Centre for Mental Health, commissioned by the National Institute for Health and Clinical Excellence. Post-traumatic stress disorder (PTSD): The management of PTSD in adults and children in primary and secondary care. Clinical guideline 26. London: Gaskell and the British Psychological Society; 2005

NHS Clinical Knowledge Summaries – Post-traumatic stress disorder www.cks.nhs.uk/post_traumatic_stress_disorder

There is a great deal of practical and highly relevant information on the provision of care for victims of torture available on the Freedom from Torture site at www.freedomfromtorture.org

Information given to candidates

> John Atto is a 42-year-old Ghanaian patient who has been registered with your surgery for 3 years.
>
> There is no medical history or clinical entries of note.

The first thing the patient says when he enters the room is, 'Hello, doctor. I've got food poisoning and need some rehydration salts and a sick note, please.'

- What do you think this station is testing?
- Make notes or discuss your thoughts with a colleague before you read on.

Plan your approach to this station:

Information given to simulated patient

Basic details – You are John Atto, a 42-year-old Ghanaian. You moved to the UK 3 years ago to work as a nurse. Your extended family lives in a village in northern Ghana and you returned from visiting them 14 days ago.

Appearance and behaviour – You have a fever and feel generally unwell. You are wearing several layers of clothes and shivering slightly because of your temperature. You are convinced you have gastroenteritis and are generally dismissive of advice you are given as you feel you know what you need.

History

Freely divulged to doctor – You feel generally unwell as you developed diarrhoea and have been vomiting for the past 3 days. You also developed a temperature 48 hours ago. You have been shivering and alternate between feeling hot and cold. You think you have food poisoning. You also have a headache, particularly when you feel hot.

Divulged to doctor if specifically asked – Your headache has worsened over the past 48 hours and is a tight band just above your eyes. You also feel generally flu-like with aching joints. You have been drinking sips of water, but if you have more than a few mouthfuls at a time you vomit. You have cramping abdominal pain when you need the toilet and the stool is watery with an unpleasant smell. There has been no blood or mucus that you have seen. You have had 6–8 loose stools per day for the past 3 days and have vomited 3–4 times over the past 24 hours. You are passing urine without discomfort but it is concentrated and also smells strongly. You are feeling thirsty. You ate the same food as your wife and friends at a restaurant in the UK last week and nobody else is unwell. You recently visited Ghana for 3 weeks, arriving back in the UK 14 days ago. This was the first time you had returned to Ghana since coming to the UK. Your family lives in a village in rural Ghana which is where you spent the majority of your visit, living in traditional mud housing. You did not seek health advice prior to travel and did not take any malaria prophylaxis. You did not use a mosquito net and were bitten by mosquitos at night on numerous occasions. You did not buy any medication while you were in Ghana.

Ideas, concerns and expectations – You think you have gastroenteritis and would like a prescription for rehydration therapy and a sick note as you are unable to work. If the doctor suggests further investigations you will say that you think these are unnecessary. You did not take malaria prophylaxis as you had malaria many times when you were living in Ghana and see it as being something you are now immune to. You were also put off by having to pay for malaria prophylaxis. You do not think hospital admission is necessary but you will agree, reluctantly, to be seen today at the hospital if it is clearly and sympathetically explained to you why this is important.

First words spoken to doctor – 'Hello, doctor. I've got food poisoning and need some rehydration salts and a sick note, please.'

Medical history – You had malaria many times when you lived in Ghana. You have no other significant medical history.

Drug history – You take no regular medications and have no drug allergies.

Social history – You live with your wife and 7-year-old son. You do not smoke or drink alcohol. You work on a surgical ward at the local hospital as a nurse. Your wife and son did not travel to Ghana with you.

Family history – Your immediate family are well and have no significant medical history.

- Having read the information given to the simulated patient, what do you now think this station is testing?
- Make notes or discuss your thoughts with a colleague before you turn the page.

Review your approach to this station:

Tested at this station:

1. Dealing with a patient with firm ideas about their diagnosis.
2. History-taking skills.
3. Physical examination skills.
4. Managing acute illness.

Domain 1 – Interpersonal skills

Dealing with a patient with firm ideas about their diagnosis

Taking a thorough history and keeping an open mind can be difficult when a patient presents with their focus on a particular diagnosis. Rather than immediately agreeing with the diagnosis offered, it is beneficial to use techniques gleaned from the various consultation models in order to ensure that both doctor and patient come away happy:

- When patients attend with a clear diagnosis and/or outcome fixed in their minds, acknowledging this is usually a helpful starting point.
- Explain that it is important to get a full history so as to make sure the appropriate treatment can be offered.
- Use open questions to explore the presenting issues. Try using phrases such as '*I can see how gastroenteritis may be one possible diagnosis, but can you tell me a little more about what you have noticed?*'
- Try to identify the patient's and your own agendas. In this instance the patient's agenda is to get the treatment he feels he needs and your agenda may be to ensure that an accurate diagnosis is made and appropriate treatment provided. You may even want to verbalize these respective agendas so that the patient understands fully your standpoint. Once identified it is then possible to work towards satisfying both these goals.

Domain 2 – Data gathering, technical and assessment skills

History-taking skills

Unless a thorough history is taken it is possible, in this station, to miss the need for further investigations and/or referral. Diagnosis is highly dependent on the quality and accuracy of information gleaned within the consultation. An awareness that individuals visiting family in developing countries are at greater risk than tourists of developing travel-related illness further aids the diagnostic process. The following information should be sought:

- Chronology of onset and pattern of fever.
- Frequency and consistency of stools.
- Evidence of blood or mucus in stools.
- Frequency of vomiting.
- Any contact with someone who has acute diarrhoea and/or vomiting.
- Any exposure to a known source of infection (possibly contaminated water or food).

- The patient's ability to eat and drink.
- Any recent antibiotics or hospital admission raising the possibility of infection with *Clostridium difficile*.
- Any recent travel abroad:
  - destination – identify all countries visited, including stopovers during travel
  - setting – whether urban or rural areas visited
  - accommodation – access to clean water and sanitation. use of mosquito bed nets
  - activities – visits to game reserves, swimming in salt or fresh water, sexual activity
  - any self-medication while abroad (e.g. over-the-counter medication bought from local pharmacies).

Physical examination skills

A focused yet thorough clinical examination would be required at this station. Fever in returning travellers can be accompanied by a variety of signs which may help guide further investigation and management. In general, the following should be assessed:

- general condition
- temperature
- pulse
- blood pressure (BP), including checking for postural drop if appropriate
- respiratory rate
- heart sounds
- breath sounds
- hydration status, including skin elasticity and mucous membranes
- evidence of rashes
- signs of jaundice or anaemia
- abdominal examination for hepatosplenomegaly
- urine for evidence of haematuria.

In this station within the 10 minutes you would be expected to take the patient's temperature, pulse, BP, listen to his chest and heart sounds, and look in his eyes (for signs of jaundice) and mouth (to see whether mucous membranes appear moist). You would also be expected to say that you wished to examine his abdomen and check a urine sample. However, you would not be expected to examine his abdomen or urine, and the examiner will hand you a card with all of the findings:

- *Temperature*   *39.4°C*
- *Pulse*   *108/min regular*
- *BP*   *108/72 mmHg with no postural drop*
- *Respiratory rate*   *14/min*
- *Heart sounds*   *Normal*
- *Breath sounds*   *Normal*
- *Skin elasticity reduced and mucous membranes not fully hydrated*
- *Urinalysis*   *Positive for ketones only*
- *Non-tender, smooth, palpable liver edge 2 cm below costal margin*

Domain 3 – Clinical management skills

Managing acute illness

It is apparent from the history and examination findings that this patient is suffering from an acute infection and is systemically unwell. Further investigations are required in order to confirm a diagnosis from a wide number of differentials and consideration should be given to where these investigations should most appropriately be conducted:

- Fever in travellers returning from malaria-endemic regions should be suspected as due to malaria until proven otherwise. If patients are systemically unwell, hospital admission would usually be advised.
- In this scenario the most appropriate course of action would be admission for urgent further assessment, as malaria is a possibility and the patient is tachycardic, has a high temperature and is showing signs of dehydration.
- In situations where admission is not required, investigations should be performed related to potential exposure. Expert advice can be sought from a variety of sources in order to help identify what investigations to arrange (see Further reading). In this station you might want to ask that if the patient refused to be admitted today, might he be prepared to wait for you to speak to one of the Infectious Diseases (ID) hospital specialists for advice?
- If he refused admission, you should explain the potential risks (including risk of death) and that this would be against medical advice, but if he was adamant, you could suggest that you organize some tests urgently, including full blood count (FBC) and thick and thin blood films for malarial parasites, urea and electrolytes (U&Es), liver function tests (LFTs), HIV and stool culture.
- You can check for information on current outbreaks and disease prevalence for areas visited using the TRAVAX website or NaTHNaC (see Further reading).

Knowledge base

Reference – Johnson V *et al.* Fever in returned travellers presenting in the United Kingdom: Recommendations for investigations and initial management. *Journal of Infection* 2009; 59(1): 1–18

The following table outlines differential diagnoses to consider in this scenario.

Malaria	• Most important potentially fatal cause of febrile illness in travellers.
	• Prevalent throughout the tropics.
	• No specific symptoms but the majority of patients give a history of fever, headache, myalgia, arthralgia and malaise.
	• Treatment should be guided by available guidelines.
Enteric fever	• Typhoid and paratyphoid are, after malaria, the most common serious tropical diseases requiring treatment in travellers returning from Asia; they are relatively uncommon in Africa.
	• Fever is almost invariable. Other symptoms and signs are non-specific, and include any or none of headache, constipation/diarrhoea and dry cough.
	• Where there is a strong suspicion of enteric fever and the patient's clinical condition is unstable, treatment should be started empirically pending blood culture results.

(Continued)

(Continued)

Rickettsiae	• Rikettsial infection is common, especially in travellers visiting game parks in southern Africa. • More than 80% of patients with *Rickettsia africae* or *R. conorii* report fever, headaches and myalgia with the classic signs of an inoculation eschar, rash and lymphadenitis seen in <50%. • The combination of an illness onset within 10 days of exposure to ticks in game parks, fever and headache with or without rash is sufficient to prompt treatment with doxycycline 100 mg twice daily.
Arbovirus infection	• There are more than 500 arthopod-borne viruses; however, only some cause disease in humans and most illness is self-limiting. • Currently the most common arboviral infections in returning travellers are dengue and chikungunya. • The spectrum of illness associated with arbovirus infection varies from mild febrile illness to dengue haemorrhagic fever or dengue shock syndrome. The latter two are rare in travellers. • Most patients with dengue can be managed as outpatients, with daily FBC to check haematocrit and platelet count. In dengue, the use of non-steroidal anti-inflammatory drugs should be avoided.
Katayama syndrome (acute schistosomiasis)	• Fresh-water exposure (usually swimming in lakes or rivers) allows cercariae released from snails to penetrate intact skin. • Symptoms and signs are non-specific but include fever, lethargy, myalgia, arthralgia, cough, wheeze, headache, urticarial rash, diarrhoea and hepatosplenomegaly. • The combination of fresh-water exposure 4–8 weeks previously, fever, urticarial rash and eosinophilia makes the diagnosis likely and empiric therapy should be given.
Leptospirosis	• *Leptospira* spp. are excreted in the urine of infected animals and humans acquire the infection through direct contact either with urine or with urine-contaminated water. • Presentation varies from mild flu-like symptoms to a severe illness characterized by haemorrhage, jaundice and hepatorenal failure (Weil's disease). • Leptospirosis classically follows a biphasic course, with an initial bacteraemic phase with 'flu-like' symptoms lasting 4–7 days, followed 1–3 days later by an immune phase characterized by fever, myalgia (especially of calves), hepatorenal syndrome and haemorrhage. • Treatment should be upon suspicion due to the non-specific nature of initial investigations. Early mild disease is generally self-limiting; penicillin and tetracycline antibiotics are thought to be effective during the bacteraemic phase.
HIV	• The possibility of acute HIV infection should be considered in all travellers presenting with fever. • The UK National Guidelines on HIV testing 2008 recommend that an HIV test should be routinely offered to all men and women who report sexual contact with individuals from high-HIV-prevalence countries.

Take-home messages

- A full travel history should include destination, setting, accommodation and activities to guide investigations.
- It is important to avoid becoming overly focused on the patient's thoughts regarding possible diagnoses.
- There are several available resources reporting on travel health and disease outbreaks.

Tasks

- Re-run the scenario with the patient planning to return to Ghana and presenting for pre-travel advice.
- Re-run the scenario with the patient refusing even to see one of the ID specialists in an urgent outpatient appointment.
- Re-run the scenario changing the presenting symptoms to fit with one of the other tropical infections covered in the InnovAiT article referenced below.

1-minute explanations for patients

- Describe the steps that can be taken to reduce the risk of illnesses caused by contaminated food and water.
- Describe the steps that can be taken to reduce the chances of being bitten by insects.
- Explain the importance and options for malaria prophylaxis.

Ideas for further revision

Seeing patients with tropical diseases is relatively rare for most UK GPs, therefore it is important to familiarize yourself with the signs and symptoms of the most serious. The e-GP resource has three useful modules covering tropical medicine. Spending time in the travel immunization clinic can also be a helpful way to familiarize yourself with which conditions are prevalent in different parts of the world.

Further reading

Johnson V *et al.* Fever in returned travellers presenting in the United Kingdom: Recommendations for investigations and initial management. *Journal of Infection* 2009; 59(1): 1–18

Jones N, Simon C. Illness in returning travellers. InnovAiT 2010; 3(5): 262–268

NaTHNaC website www.nathnac.org/pro/index.htm

TRAVAX website www.travax.nhs.uk (subscription required)

Information given to candidates

Daniel Ashton is a 32-year-old patient who has recently registered at the practice.

Last week he was seen by the practice nurse and the following was recorded on the clinical record.

- Non-smoker
- Alcohol – approximately 20 units per week
- Exercise – attends the gym 1–2 times a week
- Urinalysis – normal
- Blood pressure (BP) – 122/76 mmHg
- Height 1.75 m; weight 56 kg; body mass index (BMI) 18 kg/m^2
- Single
- Reports recent weight loss and lethargy
- Previous medical history – irritable bowel syndrome, pneumonia x 2 and shingles diagnosed in the past 12 months
- Drug history – Mebeverine; no known drug allergies

As you enter the room you are greeted by the patient. The first thing the patient says is, 'Hello, doctor. I'm here for follow-up following my new patient check as the nurse was a bit concerned about my weight.'

- What do you think this station is testing?
- Make notes or discuss your thoughts with a colleague before you read on.

Plan your approach to this station:

Information given to simulated patient

Basic details – You are Daniel Ashton, a 32-year-old accountant. You have recently registered at the practice, having moved to the area to start a new job.

Appearance and behaviour – You are casually dressed and articulate. You are anxious about your weight loss but try to mask this by joking about your symptoms.

History

Freely divulged to doctor – You have recently moved from the other end of the country to take up a new job in a large accountancy firm. The move has been pretty stressful as you have had to find a new house and get to know your new role in a short space of time. Over the past 6 weeks your irritable bowel syndrome (IBS) has been playing up and you've noticed that you've lost weight as your trousers feel a little baggy. You think you may have lost 3–4 kg.

Divulged to doctor if specifically asked – You haven't had the energy to go to the gym as often as you normally would. Your appetite is also reduced as you just don't feel like eating. You haven't really recovered your appetite after developing a chest infection which needed two courses of antibiotics about 2 months ago. Over the past 6 weeks you have had 3–4 episodes of watery diarrhoea per day. There is no blood but you do sometimes pass mucus. You have tried taking loperamide occasionally when you have an important meeting, but this doesn't seem to be helping. You are increasingly lethargic, which has coincided with the diarrhoea, and you have noticed that you're falling asleep in the early evening after a busy day at work. You have no problems getting up for work in the morning and find that although you're tired, you manage to concentrate well throughout the day. You have also noticed that since your recent chest infection you have a dry cough, which occurs mainly at night or when the air conditioning is on at work. You do not have night sweats or feel breathless. You have never coughed up blood. You have not been abroad recently.

Ideas, concerns and expectations – You think the weight loss and diarrhoea are related to a flare-up of your IBS, which you relate to the stress of your new job. You think that your recent infections have been down to a run of bad luck and have not considered the possibility of an underlying diagnosis. You expect the doctor will advise you as to what medications you can take to manage the diarrhoea. You become anxious if the possibility of HIV is mentioned, having not consciously considered this diagnosis.

First words spoken to doctor – *'Hello, doctor. I'm here for follow-up following my new patient check as the nurse was a bit concerned about my weight.'*

Medical history – Over the past 12 months you have had to see your doctor on several occasions, having had two chest infections and a bad bout of shingles affecting your upper chest. Prior to this you rarely attended the surgery. You were diagnosed with IBS around 10 months ago after developing intermittent diarrhoea and bloating symptoms. These symptoms had started following a course of antibiotics for a chest infection around 12 months ago. Stool samples and blood tests were performed, but no abnormality was found. Dietary changes helped initially and you were getting only occasional cramping pains, for which you take mebeverine. You have never had a chest x-ray.

Drug history – Mebeverine 135 mg TDS.

Social and sexual history – You live alone and are currently single. You were previously in a long-term heterosexual relationship, which ended 3 years ago. Since then you have had several short relationships with women. Although you consider yourself heterosexual, in the past when you were at university you did have a number of male sexual partners. On two occasions you got very drunk and had sex with men, once at a club and once after a house party. You can't remember much about these episodes and have tried to forget them, but if asked to remember you will say that you think that you received anal penetrative sex. You didn't use condoms on these occasions. You have never paid for sex or injected drugs, although you sometimes use cocaine when out with friends.

Family history – Nil of note.

- Having read the information given to the simulated patient, what do you now think this station is testing?
- Make notes or discuss your thoughts with a colleague before you turn the page.

Review your approach to this station:

Tested at this station:

1. History-taking skills.
2. HIV risk assessment.
3. Reaching a shared management plan.

Domains 1 and 2 – Interpersonal skills and data gathering, technical and assessment skills

History-taking skills

New patient registration checks provide a useful opportunity to review a patient's medical history. This station allows candidates to demonstrate skills in taking a focused history in order to reach a differential diagnosis which should include HIV. This should include a sexual history. However, you need to be aware that you will be raising an issue that the patient has not consciously considered and you need to be sensitive to his response. Although we have moved to try to normalize HIV testing in the UK – e.g. through routine testing of pregnant women and encouraging clinicians to offer testing opportunistically to all high-risk groups – ignorance and stigma about HIV remain.

Information on the following should be sought:

- Chronological history of symptom development. When did the diarrhoea start? When did weight loss become apparent?
- Have there been any other episodes of illness in the past? Specifically, you should consider symptoms pointing to a diagnosis of HIV or HIV-related conditions such as cough, weight loss, sweats, neurological symptoms and skin infections.
- Has the patient considered any possible underlying diagnoses for his various illnesses over the last year?

HIV risk assessment

In addition to high-risk patients (such as men who have sex with men, or black African communities living in the UK) being offered and recommended HIV testing opportunistically, the following groups should be considered at increased HIV risk, and offered and recommended HIV testing. In this station you would be expected to ascertain whether the patient falls into any of the following (relevant) categories, as part of your history-taking and HIV risk assessment:

- men who have sex with men
- female sexual contacts of men who have sex with men
- patients from an area with a high prevalence of HIV (although risk should be discussed without pre-judgement as many people in this group may be at no risk)
- patients who have had multiple sexual partners
- patients who have a history of sexually transmitted infection
- patients who have a history of injecting drug use

- patients who have had blood transfusions, transplants or other risk-prone procedures in countries without rigorous procedures for HIV screening
- patients who have been subjected to sexual assault
- patients who have a current or former sexual partner who is infected with HIV, or from an area with a high prevalence of HIV or who was an injecting drug user
- patients who may have had an occupational exposure.

Domain 3 – Clinical management skills

Reaching a shared management plan

There is a clear need to negotiate around further investigations in this patient, bearing in mind his dry cough, chronic diarrhoea, unprotected sex with men and subsequent risk of HIV. If you ask to examine the patient you will be told this is not necessary and to assume that all findings are normal (other than BMI as per the nurse's entry). Therefore, clinically there is no specific reason for inpatient investigation, but urgent stool microscopy and culture, a chest x-ray and blood tests including HIV would be expected. One of the barriers to HIV testing in primary care is the perceived need for detailed pre-test counselling. However, current guidelines state that all doctors, nurses and midwives should be able to obtain informed consent in the same way that they currently do for any other medical investigation.

Essential elements which should be discussed are as follows:

- The benefits of HIV testing for the individual:
  - A negative test can provide reassurance and reinforce safe practices to reduce the risk of subsequently contracting the virus.
  - A positive test enables the patient to receive treatment which is extremely effective in reducing HIV-related illness and death. The patient would also be in a position to take steps to reduce the risk of passing on the infection to others.
- How the results of the test will be given:
  - Ensure contact details for the patient are accurate. Check what, if any, information they are happy for you to leave on an answerphone.
  - Arrange face-to-face follow-up in order to provide the results. If the test is negative, it may be feasible to contact the patient by phone in order to pass on the result. If telephone contact is planned, it can be very difficult to ask the patient to come in if the result happens to be positive.
- Check the patient has given clear consent:
  - Patients need to be aware of and agree to the test before it is performed.
- Use the test discussion to promote safer sex with condoms.

Knowledge base

Clinical indicator for diseases for adult HIV infection (adapted from the UK national guidelines for HIV testing – see Further reading below)

	Conditions where HIV testing should be offered	AIDS-defining conditions
Respiratory	Bacterial pneumonia Aspergillosis	TB Pneumocystis
Neurology	Aseptic meningitis/encephalitis Cerebral abscess Space occupying lesion of unknown cause Guillain-Barre Syndrome Transverse myelitis Peripheral neuropathy Dementia Leucoencephalopathy	Cerebral toxoplasmosis Primary cerebral lymphoma Cryptococcal meningitis Progressive multifocal leucoencephalopathy
Dermatology	Severe or recalcitrant seborrhoeic dermatitis Severe or recalcitrant psoriasis Multidermatomal or recurrent herpes zoster	Kaposi's sarcoma
Gastroenterology	Oral candidiasis Oral hairy leukoplakia Chronic diarrhoea of unknown cause Weight loss of unknown cause *Salmonella, Shigella* or *Campylobacter* Hepatitis B infection Hepatitis C infection	Persistent cryptosporidiosis
Oncology	Anal cancer or anal intraepithelial dysplasia Lung cancer Seminoma Head and neck cancer Hodgkin's lymphoma Castleman's disease	Non-Hodgkin's lymphoma
Gynaecology	Vaginal intraepithelial neoplasia Cervical intraepithelial neoplasia Grade 2 or above	Cervical cancer
Haematology	Any unexplained blood dyscrasia, including: • thrombocytopenia • neutropenia • lymphopenia	
Ophthalmology	Infective retinal diseases, including herpesviruses and toxoplasma Any unexplained retinopathy	Cytomegalovirus retinitis
Ear, nose and throat	Lymphadenopathy of unknown cause Chronic parotitis Lymphoepithelial parotid cysts	
Other	Mononucleosis-like syndrome (primary HIV infection) Pyrexia of unknown origin Any lymphadenopathy of unknown cause Any sexually transmitted infection	

Take-home messages
- Consider HIV testing in patients presenting with conditions suggestive of the diagnosis and opportunistically in patients at high risk.
- Pre-test counselling does not need specialist input.
- Arranging face-to-face follow-up for giving test results is helpful.

Tasks

- Re-run the scenario with the patient presenting with an AIDS-defining condition.
- Re-run the scenario with the patient having been in a long-term monogamous heterosexual relationship.
- Re-run the scenario with the patient being a health professional having sustained an undisclosed needle stick injury 18 months earlier.

1-minute explanations for patients

- Explain how HIV testing is performed.
- Describe the difference between HIV and AIDS.
- Explain how HIV affects the immune system.

Ideas for further revision

The RCGP curriculum statement on sexual health recommends that GPs have skills in providing advice on safe sex and risk reduction. Specialist genitourinary medicine (GUM) services provide excellent opportunities for trainees to have expert tuition and exposure to counselling, testing and advising patients how they can protect themselves from the risk of sexually transmitted infections.

Further reading

British HIV Association, BASHH and British Infection Society. UK national guidelines for HIV testing (2008) www.bashh.org/documents/1838

e-GP module – HIV and Why early diagnosis matters www.e-GP.org

Madge, S, Matthews, P, Singh, S, Theobald, N. *HIV in Primary Care* (2nd edn) www.medfash.org.uk/publications/documents/HIV_in_Primary_Care.pdf

NICE. Increasing the uptake of HIV testing among men who have sex with men. Quick reference guide. March 2011 www.nice.org.uk/nicemedia/live/13413/53678/53678.pdf

NICE. Increasing the uptake of HIV testing among black Africans in England. Quick reference guide. March 2011 www.nice.org.uk/nicemedia/live/13417/53595/53595.pdf

Rigg, C. HIV – diagnosis and initial management. InnovAiT 2011; 4(9): 520–526

APPENDIX I

Station 1–16

Grid of stations and clinical areas covered (categories taken from GP Curriculum Statements)

Case	1 Depression; upset	2 Asthma; smoker	3 Mum re: obese son	4 Acne; wants Roaccutane	5 Erectile dysfunction	6 Otitis media; demanding	7 Complaint re colleague; diabetes	8 Hypertension	9 Dizziness	10 Glandular fever	11 Infertility	12 Crohn's disease; telephone	13 Back pain; talkative	14 Pain control; palliative	15 Feverish child; telephone	16 Domestic violence
Learn dis																
H Pro			×					×		×						
Drug use																
Psy	×				×				×							
Pall														×		
Sex					×					×						
M					×											
F											×					
Geri									×							
Paed			×												×	
Acute																
Gene																
Derm				×												
Rheum													×			×
Resp		×														
Neuro																
Endo							×									
Eye																
ENT						×				×						
GI												×				
CVD								×								

Station	Gender mix	Age mix	Skills in diagnosis	Ongoing management skills	Clinical practical skills	Health promotion	Diversity and ethical issues	Dealing with patients' emotions
Depression	F	30						×
Asthma	M	44				×		
Obese son	F (mother)	44, son 12				×		
Acne	F	23		×				
Erectile dysfunction	M	54	×					
Ear infection	F	56						×
Complaint re colleague	F	48						×
Hypertension	M	58		×				
Dizziness	F	74			×			
Glandular fever	F	16	×					
Infertility	F	20	×					
Crohn's disease – telephone consultation	F	42		×				
Back pain	F	46			×			
Palliative – home visit	M	78		×				
Feverish child – telephone consultation	F (mother)	35, daughter 2	×					
Domestic violence	F	32						×

Station 17–32

Grid of stations and clinical areas covered (categories taken from GP Curriculum Statements)

	17	18	19	20	21	22	23	24	25	26	27
Learn dis			×								
H Pro										×	
Drug use											
Psy	×										
Pall											
Sex											
M											
F								×			×
Geri	×										
Paed											
Acute						×					
Gene											
Derm											
Rheum							×				
Resp											
Neuro					×						
Endo		×									
Eye					×			×			
ENT				×							
GI										×	
CVD			×			×					
Case	17 Male carer and male partner; ?dementia	18 Thyroid disease	19 Learning disability and heart failure	20 Tinnitus	21 Visual problems in bus driver; ?MS scsclerosis	22 Chest pain; ?MI; home visit	23 Shoulder pain	24 PV discharge; interpreter	25 Wants sick note; angry	26 Dyspepsia; offensive language	27 HRT; expert patient

28	Drug misuse	×	×																	
29	Lung cancer; breaking bad news															×				
30	PTSD; asylum seeker			×																
31	Fever in returning traveller										×									
32	Weight loss; HIV risk				×															

Station	Gender mix	Age mix	Skills in diagnosis	Ongoing management skills	Clinical practical skills	Health promotion	Diversity and ethical issues	Dealing with patients' emotions
?Dementia – carer	M carer (absent patient)	72 – carer (68 – patient)					×	
Hypothyroidism	F	42	×					
Learning disabilities	F (absent patient)	50 – sister (44 – patient)					×	
Tinnitus	F	58			×			
?MS	M	32	×					
Chest pain – home visit	M	74	×					
Shoulder pain	M	58			×			
PV discharge – using interpreter	F	38					×	
Wants sick note	M	58						×
Dyspepsia	M	38		×				
HRT	F	48		×				
Drug misuse	M	20				×		
Breaking bad news	M	72						×
PTSD; asylum seeker	M	42					×	
Fever in returning traveller	M	42	×					
Weight loss; HIV risk	M	32	×					

HRT, hormone replacement therapy; PTSD, post-traumatic stress disorder; PV, per vaginal; MI, myocardial infarction; MS, multiple sclerosis.